BRAINLASH

BRAINLASH

MAXIMIZE YOUR RECOVERY
FROM MILD BRAIN INJURY

THIRD EDITION

Gail L. Denton, PhD

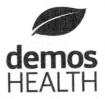

demos
HEALTH

Visit our web site at www.demoshealth.com

LIBRARY OF CONGRESS CATALOGING-IN-PUBLICATION DATA

Denton, Gail L.
  Brainlash : maximize your recovery from mild brain injury / Gail L.
Denton. – 3rd ed.
    p. cm.
  Includes bibliographical references and index.
  ISBN-13: 978-1-932603-40-8 (pbk. : alk. paper)
  ISBN-10: 1-932603-40-9 (pbk. : alk. paper)
  1. Brain damage–Popular works. I. Title.
  RC387.5.D46 2008
  617.4'8103–dc22
          2007047849

Although a great deal of care has been taken to provide accurate and current information, the ideas, suggestions, general principles, and conclusions presented in this text are subject to your personal health and sound medical advice. Every possibility is not represented, nor do we presume that all possibilities relate to your situation. This book should not be used as a substitute for recognized medical treatment modalities. Always consult your healthcare practitioner for medical advice.

For maximum benefit from the use of this book, incorporate this text in conjunction with a therapy plan through the offices of a qualified and empathetic professional physician, psychologist, neuropsychologist, or cognitive therapist knowledgeable in the field of mild traumatic brain injury recovery. This effort may include medications prescribed and monitored by your primary care physician, physiatrist, neurologist, or psychiatrist. Team effort is encouraged.

Although the vast majority of brain-injury symptoms resolve within three months, for 25% to 30% of people, the symptoms persist for two years and beyond. You may find yourself within the pages of this book. It is my great hope that you will find help, ideas, direction, courage, and support in your recovery process.

SPECIAL DISCOUNTS ON BULK QUANTITIES of Demos Medical Publishing books are available to corporations, professional associations, pharmaceutical companies, health care organizations, and other qualifying groups. For details, please contact:

Special Sales Department
Demos Medical Publishing
11 W. 42nd Street
New York, NY 10036
Phone: 800-532-8663 or 212-683-0072
Fax: 212-683-0118
E-mail: orderdept@demosmedpub.com

MADE IN THE UNITED STATES OF AMERICA

07 08 09 10   5 4 3 2 1

To Fatima, Bubba, and Mumsy,
the Black Belt Shoppers Consortium.
I owe you my life. I offer you my love.

To Mary Ann Keatley, PhD,
mentor and first champion of this book.

To M.F.K. Fisher and Susan Tweit.

I miss you, Dad.

Special thanks are extended to Daniel J. Downs, my husband,
best friend, and source of boundless unconditional love and support
throughout this project, and all its revisions. His encouragement and
devotion during my recovery are paramount to the development of this
book and its iterations. His computer skill and remarkably endless
patience with my computer struggle will forever amaze and bless me.
I love you.

This book has been written in small sections
so you can touch one piece at a time.
This book has been designed with you in mind.

JOURNAL ENTRY, APRIL 26, 1993

I am a writer.
Let me write that one more time.
I am a writer.
My heart sings when I write.
I declare this is the truth.
The next step of the path is the scribbler's step.

— Mea Culpa

SPECIAL NOTE

Dr. Denton came into my life in a most amazing way. I applied for and won a scholarship to attend a conference held by the Spinal Injury Foundation. I sat next to a therapist who asked me if I had ever read the book *Brainlash*. He explained that the author was a brilliant therapist who had sustained a brain injury and pulled herself up and out of the surrounding quagmire to write a book that brought healing to others.

I was desperate to get this book. All the major booksellers were sold out, and I finally ended up contacting the author Dr. Gail Denton. She was supportive and encouraging with practical help, and, most importantly, she had a book I could purchase. One of her practical suggestions was to get people like friends and family to tell you what they thought you could be good at. I mostly asked doctors and family because that is who I saw day after day. To my surprise they all recommended that I work toward establishing mental health and cognitive healing for others. My life and educational pursuits are now centered on bringing educational leadership to the cognitive and emotional aspects of brain injury recovery.

We can all go farther than we think we can. Sometimes others can see more potential in us than we see in ourselves. Listen to those who bring healing positive words.

— Amy Price, PhD

CONTENTS

III EXECUTIVE FUNCTIONS

IV THE TOOLBOX

V THE PHYSICAL BODY

VI THE EMOTIONAL BODY

PREFACE

Mild traumatic brain injury (MTBI) is a historically recent epidemic, gaining a foothold in modernized culture. As our lives and vehicles move faster, we play harder and our domestic relationships wear threadbare.

Acquired brain injury—prompted most widely by vehicle crashes, sports injury and domestic violence—races undetected, underdiagnosed, and undertreated through our society.

Among the medical professions (untrained to recognize it), the insurance community (unwilling to pay for adequate recovery), and the legal sector (unable to represent the loss or grasp the consequences), the mildly brain-injured individual has little to rely upon and less to go on.

MTBI is an outwardly invisible illness. External forces cause internal injury to the central nervous system. Although a direct blow to the head or face can result in brain injury, the force inflicted (whiplash, baby shaking, a twisting fall) frequently does not directly result in an external blow. Consequently, no external body marks will be evident.

The diagnosis of MTBI can be very difficult to make and may be masked or complicated by other symptoms, or "look-alike" symptoms, of other medical problems. Brain-injury research and available training in the proper diagnosis of the malady are newly emerging. Brain injury is frequently misdiagnosed as depression, panic or anxiety disorder, hypoglycemia, chronic fatigue syndrome, and even menopause. If your "brainlash" occurred without a bump on the head, the "no-blood-no foul" diagnostic approach may produce an incomplete or inaccurate picture of the situation.

The key concept here is "diffuse axonal stretching." The axon is a long single nerve-cell process (arm) that conducts nerve information impulses away from the nerve cell body to its intended destination. When internal jarring occurs, these axons are stretched out of shape and disturbed. They can no longer adequately perform their task. When the disturbed axons occur in the brain and spinal cord complex, the functions of the brain are disrupted.

Because this occurs in direct response to the mechanism of injury, and often occurs subtly, use of diagnostic tools such as MRI and CT scans fail to identify the damage. A diagnostically subtle injury, unique to each individual accident pattern, proves difficult to diagnose with today's standards of investigation.

Add to that the additional category of metabolic brain injury (anoxia, lack of oxygen to the brain), which can occur in tandem with trauma, and the plot merely thickens again.

Brainlash is written in, concise chapters that deal with specific topics pertaining to recovery from mild brain injury. As you may have noticed, the print is easier to read than in most books. It is larger, bolder, and more widely spaced. The text is also printed on paper that has a lower-than-usual glare factor to address your sensitive eyes. You may find that wearing sunglasses or placing a sheet of colored cellophane over the page will further improve your reading ability and comfort.

The short chapters are designed to fit your attention span, delivering brief, powerful aids to your healing process.

You may use this book for as little as six months or for as long as two to three years or longer. During that time, you may notice the various layers of recovery, and you may deal with the same issues repeatedly on new levels of complexity. Recovery from a brain injury is generally a longer-term experience. Two years may be a minimum length of time. You may find yourself referring back to chapters you thought you had "done."

You may wish to work very slowly and deliberately. If necessary, at first you may even wish to have someone read the book to you. This is a great way to get started. And because I encourage journaling as early as possible, taking short notes may be how you begin journaling. Dictation to another person may be your first stab at it. The key is, find a way to begin journaling.

This book benefits mildly brain-injured people who wish to know more about recovering from their injury. It assists family members, spouses, significant friends, and family acquaintances in understanding and coping with the condition of their loved one. It instructs doctors and healthcare providers in the experience of their patients, especially when the patients cannot articulate for themselves. It provides attorneys who represent brain-injured clients with a clear enumeration of the consequences, short- and long-term, of their clients' lifestyle. It enlightens health insurance companies to the struggle faced by their insured. It focuses and encourages employers to implement the options available to retain their employees. And finally, the book informs all support system members to the needs and choices available to provide optimal care and service to the brain-injured person before them.

Brainlash provides brain-injured people with an articulate interpretation of their experiences. Translating the sequela is often taxing to the individual, so the consequences of their injury are frequently left unspoken or inadequately and frustratingly misspoken. The simple act of explaining the situation causes tremendous fatigue.

I wrote *Brainlash* to make sense of my experience—and to share what I have learned along the way. I offer it as a way of understanding the depth and breadth of the road ahead for everyone involved in the process of recovery. It is my hope that your journey will be enhanced, enlightened and supported thereby.

Author's Brief Chronicle of Injury and Therapy Summary

May 1991: In-line skating accident that produced a ruptured spleen, blood loss causing anoxia, blood transfusion that rejected and lowered blood oxygen a second time, and a whiplash injury to the spine, neck, and head causing MTBI. The ultimate diagnosis was "severe" mild traumatic brain injury and anoxia. The juxtaposition of severe and mild is to me the central irony of this experience.

Initially the spleen rupture captured complete attention. As recovery from that injury resolved, the sequela of the anoxia and the previously undiagnosed MTBI ensued. Recognition of brain injury occurred six months after the injury. Testing and soft tissue therapies were begun.

Second injury, April 1992. Accidentally struck in the face in a crowded hallway. Stunned, jaw dislocated, and a return of previous symptomology. Therapy begun again.

Third injury, April 1994. Automobile crash, whiplash, resensitization of upper body and carpal tunnel pain. Therapy begun again.

Update: January 1999. Through a comprehensive and disciplined regimen of physical exercise, strength and flexibility training, nutrition, and soft tissue therapies, I am now returned to a level of activity fairly close to my pre-accident activity level. Most recently, the addition of behavioral optometry has returned another level of energy and intellectual ability. I am happy to report that I am skiing, climbing mountains, weight training, and enjoying the fiber arts. This is made possible because I continue to exercise 3 to 4 times a week, receive massage and chiropractic care regularly, eat sensibly, sleep well, and have an unconditional support system. Maintaining a "pain neutral" status requires steady, vigilant habits of self-care.

Update: June 2007. Continued maintenance allows me an active lifestyle, staying pain neutral and enjoying outdoor activities. Last several years have seen two operations involving general anesthetics. Each anesthetic use rendered me more sensitive and expanded the amount of overall cognitive recovery time. The last surgery in 2004 required 5 months of brain-injury recovery therapy to regain levels of previous proficiency. It will be paramount to work with medical staff in the future in monitoring and adjusting the application of general anesthesia and using local anesthetic when possible. Working with the anesthesiologist in advance will be crucial to cooperation and postsurgical recovery of cognitive function.

— Gail L. Denton

ACKNOWLEDGMENTS

My love and deepest thanks go out to all those who supported this project and who believe that people with mild brain injuries need to know there is information and hope for their healing process. Special thanks to all those who believed in my recovery, who supported me in my research, and who especially offered encouragement and their professional expertise to this manuscript. We shall all benefit by their trust, faith, and generosity.

Mary Ann Keatley, PhD; Mary Lou Acimovic, MA, CCC; Juliet Carpenter, MD; Rebecca Hutchins, OD; Pamela Hart, DC; Heather Campbell, PT; Genet D'Arcy, MD; Orianne Evans, DO; Rick Olson, RP; Harry Sirota, OD; Scott Zamurut, CMT; Walter Krier, CAPI; Carol Schneider, PhD; Michele Gerard, PhD; Linda Hall-Taylor, PhD; Gerri Kier; Mary Kennedy Bulick; Julie Stapleton, MD; Ann Hanks, PT; Daniel J. Downs; Peter Seaman; Linda Clark, LCSW; Susan Tweit; M.F.K. Fisher; Edvin Manniko, OD; Carolyn Tabor, CO; Trevor Hart, CMT; Donna Nikander, FNP, PCP; Arlene Hegg, MD; Jeffrey Dann, PhD; Rachel Dale, PhD; Jake Fratkin, DOM; Stephanie Neissner, PT, CMT; David Hibbard, MD; and Marilyn Coonelly, PhD.

Part I

Hi, my name is Gail, and I have a brain injury.

Gail Denton
February 21, 1996

BEGINNINGS

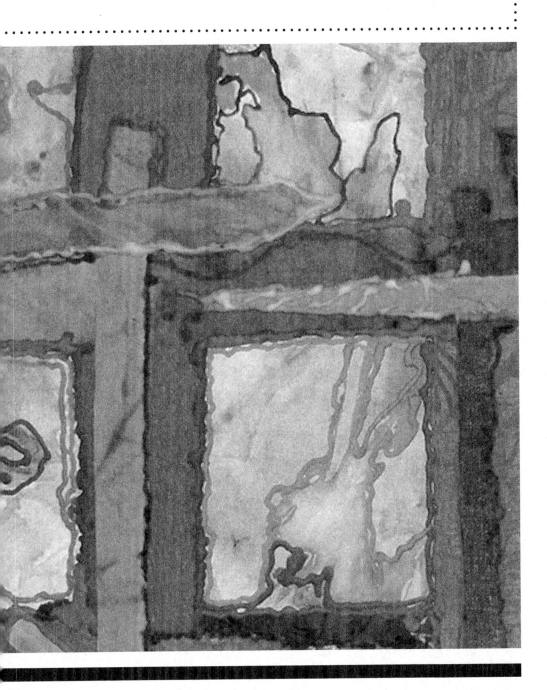

1

Introduction

It's not what happens to you
but how you respond to what happens to you
that determines the quality of your experience.

June 1992, G. Denton

On May 23, 1991, three pals went inline skating. One hit muddy grass and gravel, flipped and rolled, and ended up in the hospital. A ruptured spleen, severe blood loss, and a near-death experience followed. A week in the hospital, then three months on the couch. Slowly the anemia subsided. What remained was an underlying, undiagnosed mild traumatic brain injury.

This book records the path of my recovery. Through the twists and turns of discovery, diagnosis, treatment, experiential therapy, and emergence with a new life, the writing of this book is as much about the journey as the journey itself.

During this time, I rehabilitated, grew stronger, met and married my present husband, changed careers, wrote this book and grew to love the new person I have become as a result of the accident.

An extra thank you to my husband, Dan, who has been unconditionally by my side throughout this whole adventure.

JOURNAL ENTRY: JANUARY 15, 1993

I wrote down what I was going through in order to trace my progress, to nurture my feelings of abandonment, and to try and make sense of a journey I had never thought to take or to even/ever prepare for.

A journey of the mind. The road to recovery for mild brain damage, without so much as a bump on the head as a clue. A piece of the accident caused in part, it has been postulated, by the force of the blow to my abdomen (and the consequent Jell-O-like brain smashing into the inside of my skull because of the twisting nature of the fall—an internal whiplash) and the loss of oxygen to certain "less critical" parts of my brain due to heavy blood loss.

But because I wasn't a vegetable—because it wasn't catastrophic—because with my loss of brain power I still scored above average on the tests—they shrugged, patted me on the head, and told me to come back in two years for another test so they could measure my recovery.

Two years can be a long time if your life is upside down, your personal mortgage banker lacks a similar sense of humor, and you probably need to make your way in the world between now and then.

I guess I'm angry. Not that Western science doesn't know what to do. They seem to know what to do for the catastrophically impaired.

I've been a therapist for 15 years, and I don't remember ever telling someone to come back in two years so I could test their progress. No hints. No guidance. No clue.

"Your brain will generally gain maximum recovery in two years. Come back and we'll see how you do." And, by the way, your insurance company doesn't cover this neuropsychological test unless you have a prescription from the neurologist. Through some interesting loophole in the policy, the test is considered on the "psychology" side rather than the neurology side. A thousand dollars so someone can tell you what you've fairly well figured out for yourself in the first place or you wouldn't have gone to the neurologist.

Can't follow conversation, can't track sequential ideas, notice visual blind spots, can't tell jokes, laugh at jokes late, can't follow directions, can't add a short stack of numbers (like in the grocery store), get lost on the way to the office, don't recognize people, can't remember names, can't problem solve, cry at the drop of a hat, sex doesn't seem to work somehow, fail at following conversation and discussions with any sort of integrated or sequential theme, can't learn new information, need a map to go anywhere, blurt out inappropriate comments, overly sensitive to everything, get easily confused, very short attention span, lists and sticky notes become my daily lifesaver, get confused in traffic, can't recall details of my kids' lives, doubt my unimpaired intellect too, forget to rinse the shampoo out of my hair (it's a sequencing thing).

We called it my lumbar brain (should be limbic brain—a little anatomy humor). Journaling the changes seemed to build a trail of proof that I was healing.

But the abandonment by my own profession infuriated me. How was I supposed to get from here to two years from here without any help? They looked blankly at me and suggested I return in two years. My injury wasn't very bad. I'd gradually get better to the extent of my potential (whatever that was) in that amount of time. I could pull myself up by my bootstraps (if I could find them), or do nothing, and my brain would or wouldn't get better. Thank you very much.

I postulated that if I could heal a broken leg, an ovarian cyst, and an 8-inch scar down the middle of my belly, those same principles had to apply to my brain.

Operating as a therapist was tough going. All the skills I needed to do my job were impaired. The listening, tracking, sequencing, and problem solving were mentally exhausting. But learning a new trade was out as well.

A PhD, with 20 years of business experience, 15 years of therapist experience, and nowhere to go. Trapped and abandoned. I went to nontraditional healing systems to seek new answers. Some answers existed in acupuncture, nutrition, herbs, visualization, behavioral optometry, cross-crawling, massage, cranial sacral manipulation, polarity therapy, chiropractic, psychological kinesiology, hypnosis, Pilates, astrology, and psychic energy work. The world of subtle energy science was of great value. I threw the non-Western book at myself. Did I gain more function than if I'd eaten pizza and watched MTV for two years? Who's to know?

I do know that my quality of life was improved, if simply because I felt active in my own recovery. If I thought anchovy milkshakes would have helped, I'd have drunk them, just for the pro-active benefit.

Head-injury support groups were not for me. I didn't want to be a cliché. "How many Boulderites does it take to screw in a light bulb? Eight. They meet at dusk, form a support group, and learn to live with the darkness." I wasn't badly impaired.

My impairment is known as "highly functional minimal loss." On the grand scale, I still had more marbles in my bag than most unimpaired folks, which is nice, I suppose. But it doesn't account for my loss. Discounts my loss, actually. I'm somewhere on the bell curve outside the sympathy line.

But *I* notice the loss. No, I *live* with the loss. I used to be smarter. I used to be a doctor. Now I'm a low-spark doctor. And I remember who I used to be and how I performed. There is devastating loss here for me.

Who am I now? Where do I go from here? No map. No compass. No help. Not exactly caught in a creative moment. Not exactly equipped for self-extrication. Not exactly sure who I am, where I can go, who I'm going to be later, or what I'll do if I get where I'm going, wherever that is.

Feeling ethically challenged about going to the office, sitting under the shingle of my former self, charging big bucks, crossing my fingers, and hoping that no one runs screaming out the door, down the hall into the arms of one of the conveniently located barristers on the third floor.

A pain came with the vacuum that was the treatment model from Western medicine. No answers, and the condescending attitude really infuriated me. That iconoclastic attitude of "owners of the knowledge" combined with "kindly take your silly little problem down the hall" and don't bother us. It's all a tacky cover-up for a lack of answers, yet the need to own the territory nonetheless. Arrogance.

Arrogance is not an answer, a direction, or a therapy. Arrogance is not the truth. It is despicable, disrespectful, and inexcusable. I fought back. I will continue to take responsibility for my health. To look for additional answers to questions. To try and work out new ways to grow, change, and heal.

We all have an inner voice to guide us, whatever volume yours happens to be. Listening to it is good. Following the advice is better still.

Pieces of me will be different. Other pieces of me are gone. New pieces of me are emerging. Discovering the new nooks and crannies is a frustrating, fascinating journey. Mourning what's gone, welcoming what's new (even if it's the newest cowlick on the top of my head; if Alfalfa can make it charming, so can I).

Learning to love myself, today, each day, seems to be the final key to it all. Emerging from the pain, passing into the pleasure of this new being. "Space, the final frontier."

THE ART OF GRACEFUL RECOVERY, AUGUST 1993

Remember that you want to get well and all your physical, emotional, and mental energy is focused to that end.

You shall prevail with love for yourself in a graceful, supportive manner.

Challenge exists for us today.

We improve daily, even in minute ways that reveal themselves slowly.

We heal daily.

It feels awkward, embarrassing, undignified, and devaluing to have this invisible struggle inside me.

I want my life back.

Notice you are alive, if slightly altered and inconvenienced.

This is a good place to start.

— *G. Denton*

That Moment of Recognition

I remember that first moment of recognition, that moment I suspected, ever so briefly, that there was something wrong with my brain. It was a wide gulf of silence. Wanting to reach the other side, yet dreading the answer if I did. Knowing the consequences of my discovery. No, no, anything but that. Then the next steps after denial began to lead down a path toward seemingly endless therapy and struggle.

Let me guide you through some of those twists and turns. I can't promise to get you all the way home, but I can offer reasonable tips along the journey. Mostly, this book will endeavor to keep you from falling through the cracks: the jungle of the medical, legal, and insurance worlds. It will provide you with signposts designed to cue you to take your own action on your behalf.

So, let us begin the journey, you and I, with the cadre of pals, team members, and supporters you bring with you. Wear your good boots and bring your lunch and plenty of water. We could be out there for awhile.

The Journey Begins

What happens when frustration sets in? Does your brain shut down, do your eyes defocus, do tears well up, and does "Why me?" pour from your throat? Frustration comes with the territory. There will be days when it takes forever to go nowhere. A rough day. I called them bad brain days. There were plenty of days I sat and stared. Finally, thankfully, I came to realize that sitting and staring was a part of the healing process and not a bad thing at all.

The healing brain needs an incredible amount of rest or nonactivity to repair itself. If you try to work or think too hard when your brain wants to repair, the brain will shut you down. If you rest or nap (cooperate), then you will get clear time later. If you resist, your brain function will continue to spiral downward until you feel like you've been bound to the earth by Lilliputians.

If your brain shuts off while reading this book, please cooperate. Put a marker in the book, and come back later. We are in this together for the long haul. The book will be here when you get back, ready to support you in your healing process, for as long as you can work the next time. And the time after that.

I support you in your recovery. Writing this book helped bring me back. If, in your journey through it, you make discoveries of activities, processes, nutrients, coping strategies, exercises, or medicinal applications that are working for you, record them in your journal. You are not alone. Your journaling experiences can help you as well as others. You may find a puzzle piece that helps others, as surely as it has helped you. Let your healthcare professional know what you have discovered.

Write in your journal the things you see about yourself in this book and how the strategies have helped you. The support I received by sharing my discoveries with my friends, family members, and healthcare providers was of great value to all involved. As my support system extended a hand to me so that I could reach my bootstraps even when I couldn't remember where they were, so I offer this journal concept to allow that same support to extend to you.

Support

You need support and help, especially if you are not used to asking for support and help. Make sure you read the chapter on support, and resolve the ego battle inside yourself. It is vital to your recovery.

Small Tasks

Any task can be broken into smaller bits. If you feel overwhelmed by a task, chop it up into smaller pieces. Laundry is a classic example of a complicated task that can be subdivided. Use several baskets, and label them in the categories you use most often. At my house, the categories are lights, darks, delicates, and colors. When washing time comes, just wash one basketful. It's presorted already. (More on laundry later.)

Remember, you can always ask for help when making jobs smaller. Break the jobs up during the day. I frequently ask my husband to advise me on evaluating tasks, their importance, and their priority. Often a task can be reprioritized, handed off to others, chopped up, or even thrown off the list. Be gentle with yourself.

Not Everything Happened to Me

Most of the experiences in this book are a part of my experience. Yet there are a few areas of brain injury that I did not personally experience. Those chapters include information gathered from other brain-injured people and the experience of various cognitive therapists who consulted with me on this project. Not everything discussed in this book needs to have happened to you either. Some chapters may not apply to you. That's great! Just move on to a chapter that does apply. Remember, however, that, a year from now, a chapter you skipped may be useful. Feel free to read it later.

Postconcussive Syndrome, Mild Brain Injury

"While most persons who experience a mild brain injury notice that their cognitive symptoms (slow processing, fuzzy thinking, attention and concentration problems) disappear within three months, between 25 and 30 percent continue to have difficulty. Sometimes the problems become more obvious as people return to work or school, or when physical injuries no longer predominate.

There may be no physical evidence of the damage that is causing deficits, but they are no less real just because they do not show up on a CAT scan or an MRI. Movies and TV would have us believe that we jump up and are just fine after a brain injury, but often it takes time to recover. The brain is a very sensitive organ responsible for everything we do. When its functioning is disrupted by an injury, numerous symptoms may result."[1]

Form a Support System

When possible, use this book within a team approach that includes your primary care physician, your cognitive therapist, and other healthcare, legal, or professional team members appropriate for your situation and goals.

The Truth Is No Excuse

It's tacky but true. Some folks will use the symptoms of brain injury for personal gain through what is known as "secondary gain syndrome." For some reason, identification with brain injury is a good excuse not to return to life. Or, to get funding from insurance companies and lawsuits, there may be the temptation to "maintain" one's symptoms in order to satisfy the intricacies of legal case settlements. Personally, I can't think of a reason to pretend to have a brain injury.

Whatever the real world may hold for you, do not postpone your healing process. Protect yourself by journaling. With a daily journal (See the chapter Journaling), you can record your difficulties and improvements, your challenges and triumphs. Your journal will keep track for you. As always, consult your attorney for formal legal advice. Legal settlements can take just as many years as a longer-term recovery. The truth of your injuries is no excuse for postponing their repair. Document your recovery.

The Index

Use the index. It contains the words, phrases, and concepts contained in the text of the book. The index has been heavily cross-referenced. Find what you are looking for in the index.

Bibliography and Resource Guide

Lists of books, as well as suggested resources, organizations, and products, are found in the back of this book.

Thoughts on the Third Edition

Living with and continuing to recover from my injuries, now for more than 15 years, I have observed the status of brain-injured people and the medical and institutional responses to their various needs. One thing has become clear to me. There is a definite need to separate the response, diagnosis, and treatment approach of the "mildly injured" constituency from that of the "moderately and severely injured" constituency.

For one thing, the needs of the "mild" group are remarkably different from those of either the "moderate" or the "severe." Different treatment protocols, different levels of restorable functioning, different levels and topics of research, different functional and effective modalities, different successful treatment complexes, and different potential outcomes.

Also, I believe that the "severe" constituency, and in many ways rightly so, garner the bulk of the funding, research, and heroic response that allopathic (Western) medicine provides so well.

Because of this very need, the "mild" group gets the short end of the funding stick. Their needs are more evenly met with noninvasive, case-managed team effort—consistently applied integrative therapies in a strong combination with allopathic therapies. "mild" persons have a fairly "normal" social appearance. We blend in. We look just fine.

The time has come for mild traumatic brain injury to feature itself separately; identify its specific and unique needs, goals and client base; and gain a clear voice. Our needs are specific. We can differentiate ourselves, our needs, our organizations, foundations, research, effective treatment modalities, and recovery options and successes.

Thank you for my soapbox moment.

2

Questionnaire

*"...looking for the bruise on your brain
that no one can see..."*

G. Denton

his questionnaire will help focus your symptom discovery for brain injury. When answering these questions, do so in light of how you are presently functioning.

1. Have you been in an accident recently, say, within the last year?
2. Did you hit your head? Were you shaken, or did you experience a physical impact?
3. Were you taken to the hospital?
4. What was your diagnosis?
5. What doctors are you currently seeing?
6. Were x-rays, MRI, or CT scan taken? SPECT scan?
7. What medications are you currently taking? Were you given a prescription for this event?

Please read this list and indicate any problems you may be having. Remember to distinguish and notice if you had the problem or condition before the accident when evaluating if you have the condition presently. Note if it made a pre-existing issue worse. Rate your problems on the following scale: Never, Occasionally, Sometimes, Frequently, or Always.

PAIN

1. Do you have more headaches since your injury? Pain in the temples or forehead?
2. Do you have pain in the back of your head? Does it move forward? Are there moments of very sharp or stabbing pain that lasts for a few moments?
3. Do you tire more easily, either mentally or physically? Does fatigue worsen with pressured thinking or emotional situations?
4. Are your neck and shoulders beginning to hurt? Tingling down your arms? Overall aching feeling? Overall pain upon waking in the morning?
5. Are you overly sensitive to light, sound, motion, or intense environments? Do you have dark spots before you eyes or blurred vision? Does it get worse with fatigue?

MEMORY

1. Do you lose or misplace items?
2. Do you forget what people tell you? Or what you have said to others?
3. Do you forget where you parked your car? Or your current driving destination?
4. Do you forget what you've read? Or the last TV or radio topic?
5. Are you having difficulty remembering life details from the past?

ATTENTION AND CONCENTRATION

1. Are you having trouble concentrating? Holding a thought?
2. Do you have difficulty concentrating in noisy or strongly lit environments?
3. Do you have difficulty concentrating on more than one topic or task at a time?
4. Do you have difficulty focusing your attention while reading or watching TV?
5. Are you having difficulty staying focused when you are driving?
6. Do you have difficulty making decisions? Or remembering what you decided?

7. Do you drift off in conversation, unable to recall what has been said?

8. Is it stressful to read and answer this questionnaire?

9. Are you easily distracted? When interrupted, do you struggle to find your place again or return to your task?

10. Have you become impulsive, making decisions or remarks without thinking them through? Unintentionally hurting someone's feelings? Impulse shopping?

LANGUAGE AND COMMUNICATION

1. Do you have difficulty following a conversation?

2. Do you have difficulty thinking of the exact word or words you want to use?

3. Do you have problems expressing yourself in writing?

4. Is it difficult conversing with others or staying in a conversation?

5. Are you struggling to spell words? Do you reverse the letters?

6. Are you pronouncing words correctly? Is your tongue twisting words around or relocating words inaccurately in a sentence?

VISUAL PERCEPTION

1. Do you have increased sensitivity to light, sound, shopping, party, or large meeting environments?

2. Do objects seem closer or farther away than they actually are?

3. When reading, do printed letters appear to change their shape or position on the page? Are you experiencing eye strain or headaches when reading?

4. Do you have difficulty focusing your eyes on objects?

5. Do you feel dizzy or nauseous? Are you bumping into objects more than usual? Whacking your elbows, hitting your head, or stubbing your toes frequently?

6. Do your eyes struggle to track written text or follow moving objects?

EXECUTIVE FUNCTION

1. Do you have difficulty following through with planning for work or leisure activities? Do you accurately gauge the time a task will take?

2.   Do you have problems setting goals and priorities and keeping to your plan?

3.   Do you have difficulty starting new tasks? Does a new task trigger depression, hopelessness or fatigue? Do you struggle to get in the mood to begin?

4.   Do you have difficulty monitoring and correcting your errors?

5.   Do you have difficulty changing from one task to another?

6.   Are you able to anticipate the consequences of your actions? Can you foresee outcomes or project the future of a task.

7.   Are you checking and rechecking your work? Does the slightest disruption in your routine derail you?

8.   Are you unintentionally repeating yourself in conversation?

EMOTIONAL FUNCTION

1.   Have you noticed frequent mood swings or emotional outbursts?

2.   Do you have difficulty handling your anger?

3.   Do you feel depressed? Are you fearful? Have you lost hope? Are you tired of fighting for recovery? Just want your life back the way it was?

4.   Do you have feelings of anxiety, jumpiness, or nervousness?

5.   Do family and friends comment on changes in your behavior? Are people living around you on the outskirts of you?

6.   Trouble sleeping? Poor appetite or binge eating? Craving stimulant foods?

7.   Do you feel hopeless, although you can identify things that are hopeful or positive? Does hope feel just out of your reach?

8.   Have you become gullible? Easily distractible or unintentionally naïve? Can you tell when you are being teased, and do you respond with humor?

9.   Are you easily startled, agitated, or irritated? Do you respond with aggression? Feel tense or wound up all the time? Overly sensitive to your environment?

FINANCES AND MEASUREMENTS

1.   Do you have difficulty easily performing simple addition and subtraction?

2.   Can you easily make change at the store?
3.   Do you struggle to balance your checkbook as accurately as before?
4.   Do you remember to open your mail, sort it, and pay your bills on time?
5.   Can you follow a recipe easily, or comprehend and follow instructions to assemble or operate something? Can you easily follow a map or directions to a location?

ORGANIZATION AND SEQUENCING

1.   Do you have difficulty following the steps of a recipe?
2.   Do you attend to your mail on a regular basis? Can you accurately sort the junk mail and focus on mail worthy of your time and energy?
3.   Do you struggle with performing, initiating, or keeping up with normal, routine household chores?
4.   Do you have difficulty performing more than one household task at a time?
5.   Can you effectively manage your time? Do you lose track of time?
6.   Do you set priorities and fulfill your obligations?
7.   Do you follow through on a project to the end, or do you set it aside with good intentions, yet ultimately abandon it?

SAFETY

1.   Do you forget to turn off the iron, stove, tea pot, or other household appliances?
2.   Do you forget where you are going when driving your car?
3.   Do you forget to lock your doors at home? Do you lock your car doors? Garage door?
4.   Do you forget important appointments (e.g., picking up the kids, going to your doctor's appointment, banking your paycheck)?
5.   Do you feel like your safety awareness levels are less than they should be?
6.   Has your tolerance for alcohol, caffeine, or drugs decreased?

LIFESTYLE

Other quick questions you may relate to include: (Answering *Never, Occasionally, Sometimes, Frequently,* and *Always*)

○ Remembering where your keys, glasses, purse, wallet are?

○ Remembering to brush your teeth, eat breakfast, and shower?

○ Remembering how to do all the parts of your job?

○ Do you lose track of time? Forget to eat? Forget who you just dialed on the phone?

○ Are you sleeping well? Are you easily fatigued?

○ Do you feel overwhelmed, or unable to cope?

○ Are you intolerant of noise? Even traffic noise? Even the dishwasher?

○ To have a successful conversation, must you turn off the radio or TV first?

○ Are you restless? Do you worry more? Lack patience?

○ Are you overwhelmed by simple pleasures, or by people you used to enjoy?

○ Do you feel like you are "losing it?" Out of control? Going crazy?

○ Do you hopelessly search for the word you want?

○ Is your speech slurred or jumbled? Are you inventing words that get jammed into each other?

○ Is your body's temperature in control? Your appetite?

○ Are there changes in your sex drive or sexual response? Is orgasm a struggle?

○ Are there changes to your menses? Your sleep cycle? Digestive rhythm?

Likely, you see yourself in these questions. Somehow, your brain and emotional functions are different than they were before your incident. You need to know that you are not alone, and you are not crazy. There are actions you can take to enhance your mending process and to maximize your brain's opportunity to recover and function to its highest potential.

Part II

LIFE ISSUES

"…butter side down…"
Murphy's Law

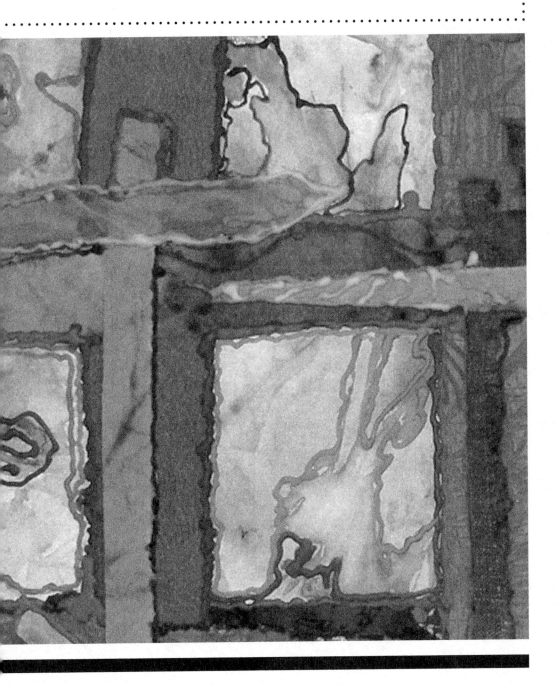

3

Lifestyle Changes and Challenges

Your reorganized and newly evolving lifestyle plan:

Brain injury often brings with it a shift in lifestyle. Employment may dwindle or vanish. Health insurance may not cover the needed therapies. Finances crumble, life seems outside your control, relationships shift and emotions wash over the entire depressing scene. The future is a maze that your brain struggles to solve and comprehend.

There will be lifestyle changes, challenges, and adjustments. This chapter will help you navigate these new and temporary adjustments and will support your therapeutic process.

Money

Let's get right to the point. If you can't think, you can't work. If you can't work, you can't pay the bills. This is a very straightforward issue.

What happens when financial devastation, or what looks and feels like it, is staring you in the face? What do you do? What can you do?

Keeping perspective in this situation is very important. You may not be able to work just now. Or you may be able to work a little or a medium amount. Discover your performance level and do not exceed it. (See the chapters "Attention Span and Overwhelm" and "Relapse" for information on overdoing it.)

Your expectations will change, your goals will change and your deadlines will change. For a while, your lifestyle will be altered. Your ability to take care of yourself will decrease. For a time, your brain will give you what it can to survive, and that may be all you get.

Your job is to determine what you are given by your brain to "fund" your life and then to live within that budget. Ideas and strategies for figuring all this out are found in subsequent chapters.

Downsizing Your Lifestyle

To that end, you must downsize your daily life activities, expectations, and budget to fit your brain "allowance." Temporarily, you are on a nonnegotiable budget, an allocation over which you have no control. The sooner you realize this and cooperate, the sooner your energy will be used for living and healing.

Of course, because of your injury, perspective and budgets, plans and deadlines, and outlines and finances maybe outside your thinking ability. This is a great time to ask for help and support from someone you trust. Generally, that person is your accountant or bookkeeper, your partner, or a family member. Choose someone who is organized, can balance a budget, and has a sense of the "big picture." Be prepared to explain to them why you need help and how it is that they can specifically assist you. Remember, because your brain injury is invisible, your need for help is not obvious.

Keep reminding yourself that this is temporary. The stress caused by drastically altered finances can sap your energy supply. Ask for help.

The KISS Principle

Keep it simple (KISS) when downsizing your lifestyle. Cut back or eliminate activities that you cannot afford or for which you have no energy or time. Let go of volunteer activities. Either call the organizations and withdraw your services without further notice, or have a friend call for you (if saying "no" is a part of your challenge). Take a leave of absence. That is your truth. Learn to "just say no." Your life is overwhelming. Let go of these activities for now.

What About My Job?

It is entirely likely that you will not be able to work at all, at first. Over time, you may be able to return for half days, part-time, flex-time, and even full-time. Depending upon your rate of recovery, this process could take three months or three years. There is a slim chance that you will be able to work only part time even after three years.

This may be a serious financial reality for you. Yet, it is imperative that you not rush the healing process by returning to work beyond your ability level. Ultimately, your decision to return to work could alter the healing process and keep you exhausted, stressed out, and unable to improve your health.

Depending on the nature of your occupation, returning to work early may endanger the lives of others, cause unnecessary errors, and potentially jeopardize your professional future. You also may not be ready to drive your car. (See "Driving.")

Consult the chapter "Work" for more information on returning to the jobsite and for handy tips and exercises on how to maximize your return-to-work experience.

Therapy Time

The time you used to spend going to work may likely be taken up now with going to therapy. With an active recovery program, you may end up seeing therapists of one sort or another several times a week. Early on in my therapy, I saw a massage therapist twice a week, a chiropractor once a week, an acupuncturist once a week, an exercise/walking buddy twice a week, a psychotherapist once a week, and an Aston Patterning physical therapist once a week. Years later, I still include weekly massage therapy, weekly eye therapy, almost daily exercise, and a chiropractic appointment every couple of weeks.

Just going to therapy can be exhausting and can require several hours of recovery afterward. For the first six months, I just went to therapy, then home to rest and integrate the information.

The second six months, after the acute physical pain was reduced, I began to add in more exercise time and fewer soft tissue therapies. Cognitive therapies entered the picture. But, still, therapy took up a good 10 to 12 hours of each week (plus driving time).

Insist that your healthcare providers cooperate in creating a reasonable schedule of appointments for you. Ask them to piggyback appointments so that you get at least one day a week away from appointments. Just getting to and from appointments can be exhausting. Cluster them whenever possible. Strive for efficiency.

If your injury does not involve serious soft tissue injury as well, this time commitment may be decreased. Do not be surprised, however, if your combined therapies take center stage in your schedule for a year or more. Be sure to inform your therapist if your drive to the appointment has exhausted you. It is wise to select a more gentle regime for that session.

The Cost of Therapy

Make sure that your diagnosis is fully covered by your health plan and that your insurance company understands the nature of your injuries. You may have to consult an attorney. Do not hesitate to consult an attorney if your insurance company does not honor the diagnosis and treatment prescribed by your attending healthcare provider. BE WARY OF ANY OFFER FOR EARLY CLAIM SETTLEMENT.

You may not know the full extent of your condition for several years, or the full range of therapies needed to support your recovery. Be wary of an early payoff offer. Consult an attorney before accepting any kind of settlement from your insurance company or (in the case of an auto crash in which you were not at fault, for instance) the insurance company of any other involved party.

Your insurance company can get a second opinion from one of its privately selected doctors at any time (the IME, independent medical examination). This sort of situation can generally be avoided if your healthcare team diligently provides treatment plans with objective goals and office notes to back up each treatment session. When this paperwork is systematically provided to your insurance company, decisions are then made from a more informed point of view. It is a style of care that works well for both the insurer and the insured.

Legal Advice

Attorneys give legal advice, and that is what you may need. Generally, the specialty of attorneys in these cases is called personal injury and is usually found as a sub header in the yellow pages under *Attorney*. If you cannot find it, ask the local Bar Association for a referral based upon the nature of your case.

Interview at least three attorneys before selecting one. This is almost like selecting a best friend. You will need a professional who is knowledgeable in brain-injury cases, not just generic personal injury. Select someone to whom you can relate, and from whom you will receive respect. If possible, request referrals from the attorneys of previous clients who have had brain injuries.

Not everyone will need an attorney. There are excellent health insurance policies and excellent insurance companies as well. Sometimes brain-injury cases are the true test of the strength of your policy. Healing from a long-term injury, such as brain injury, takes time and funding. Make sure someone in your support system understands your policy and can deal with the insurance company for you, should the need arise. (See the chapter, "Support Systems".)

Television

During recovery, believe it or not, your television can be useful. Unless you never watch it, or do not own one, it can be a therapeutic tool. First of all, your brain will need "vegetation time" during waking hours. Not all brain rest takes place during sleeping or napping. Either staring off into space or staring off at a television can accomplish the same thing: brain rest. It is a way to offer your brain wakeful rest.

On the other hand, for some people, television time saps energy and must be severely limited. You may not be ready for it. If you find that you are either too engaged by programs or that you are more tired or emotionally agitated than before you sat down to watch, television time may not be appropriate. Turn the darned thing off! Especially avoid violent programs, the news and tawdry topics.

For most of us, the television can also be a therapeutic tool for cognitive rehabilitation. Some, but certainly not all, programming can remind us of what we know, triggering thought patterns and memory.

If you are a soap opera fan, following along with all the juicy little subplots can trigger sequencing, memory, and attention span. If you are a current events buff, then CNN may be your cup of tea. For data recovery, Jeopardy is excellent. For puzzles, Wheel of Fortune fills the bill. Game shows are great for trivia recall. They remind you of what you know and assist in self-esteem recovery.

Talk shows can be useful too. I found Oprah and Donahue especially helpful because they were always interviewing healthcare professionals. I could find professional triggers back to my knowledge base. Later in recovery, the McNeil-Lehrer Report refreshed my political brain and helped me think more complex thoughts.

Old movies are therapeutic because they tend to dwell on character development, plot, and substance. Old movies are heavy on message and light on violence. (Violent programming can be overwhelming.)

Rocky and Bullwinkle cartoons, the Saturday mornings of my childhood, made me laugh and reminded me of happier times. Excellent for memory and pleasure.

Renting videos, or borrowing from the vast library of a friend, increases your viewing possibilities. Old Star Trek episodes are worth a try, too.

If you have cable or satellite access, the comedy channels can also be a source of entertainment, as well as stimulation for the brain to engage in complex reasoning.

Humor

Sense of humor is a very complex, personal, subtle, and sequenced skill. You may discover that you do not "get" jokes for a while: those told to you or those played on you. You may lose your ability to tell jokes. This can be a very sad discovery, especially if your personality once incorporated humor, or you were just naturally funny or creatively insightful. Humor will take a while to return.

When listening to a joke that you do not understand, ask someone to explain the punch line to you. It's a good form of external modeling. Try to repeat the joke you heard. Learn another joke and try repeating it. Hang in there. (See the chapter, "Humor.")

Weight Gain and Weight Loss

One of the results of reduced physical activity may be weight gain. It could be the result of biochemical messages from the brain as extra psychological protection from your environment. The appetite message gets confused and the brain forgets to say "stop eating."

It could be that recreational eating has caught up with you now that you have reduced your activity level.

Biochemical depression, present in most people with brain injuries, can also cause carbohydrate and chocolate cravings, which lead to love handles.

Weight loss may also occur if you deal with depression or inactivity associated with a loss of appetite. The brain can also be in biochemical imbalance and forget to tell you to eat. You may not perceive that you are hungry and have no craving for food. Awareness is important here. (See the chapter, "Depression.")

Control of Your Life

One of the first things that can depart from your life with brain injury is a feeling of control over events, emotions, and the people around you. This is a reasonable response to your circumstances.

Your world is suddenly different, and gaining control of it again may be a puzzle you cannot solve just now. Gaining control of your life again is a new long-term goal. Losing control of your life was not on your agenda.

This journal entry frames my feelings.

AUGUST 4, 1992

Money and midlife crisis. Now there's the wicked couple, if ever. Either you got a lot of it and paid too high a price, or you're not where you "thought" you'd be by now.

And even though money isn't everything, it does cover the mortgage and the orthodontist bill, so let's not play any yuppie creation games with money. Money isn't really the point anyway. Happiness is. Even the black-belt shoppers can't buy happiness.

But since you want it and don't have it, why is that?

Which dream did you purchase that left you elsewhere when you looked up the other day? Some incredible externally identified movie that had a cost, and a destination. You paid the price, you didn't get there, and the salesman hasn't been seen in these parts for many moons.

So here you are. Re-examining your purchase. Does it still fit? Are you where you were promised? Do you even want to still go there? Could be a perfectly reasonable destination, but you may have changed your mind. Buyer's remorse.

Gaining control will come slowly. With each discovery and gain in your new life, control may look different than it used to. Be open to new ways to express control in your life. It will soften the impact of the journey.

It is important to determine what aspects of your life are actually within your control. Get help acting on those aspects. Then ask someone about the aspects of your life over which you need to regain control. Finally, what aspects do you need to have the serenity to accept as presently out of your control? In many ways, gaining that control is just as important as establishing what you can control and what is beyond your grasp at the moment. Be at peace with your answers.

Support Systems

It is entirely likely that you will need help in your life during recovery. Suddenly, what used to be second nature (like fixing a bowl of cereal) becomes an exhausting ordeal. You will probably need help with the daily routine of life.

Suddenly, cleaning the house, shopping, driving, cooking, and paying bills—even fetching the mail or the newspaper from the curb—are overwhelming tasks. You may have days when none of these get done. Petting your cat may be the activity of the day—and then only if the cat jumps into your lap.

There are three major components to the process of support: (1) identifying the job, (2) asking for help and (3) accepting help.

Your family, your friends, and especially your spouse or significant other are all available to help, on some level. Since you may not look sick, they may not know that you could use a hand. You must ask for support. Learn more about how to do that effectively by reading the chapter on "Support Systems."

Emotions

The biochemical changes that occur with some brain injuries can also generate mood swings, depression, withdrawal, and a rollercoaster ride that feels like it may never end. Add that to pre-existing life events like midlife crisis, menopause, marriage, or graduation, and you have a recipe for an amusement ride for which Disney would pay good money.

You may feel like a slave to your emotions. You may feel blindsided, bushwhacked, ambushed, and held captive by aliens who make you act in ways that are unfamiliar to your experience. And yet, there you are. Brain injury can add to as well as subtract from your repertoire of behaviors. (See the chapters "New Abilities and New Skills" and "Emotions and Denial.")

Knowing that emotional distress and spontaneous behaviors happen to most brain-injured people is small consolation. When you are the one throwing cereal boxes in the grocery store, there is no other world. When the minister asks a rhetorical question and you stand up and answer it in front of the whole congregation, it seems perfectly logical. At the time.

When tears stream down your face, for any reason, your life can feel bigger than before. Emotions will be different. The chapter "Self-Esteem" will help you remember to love yourself during this interesting part of recovery. Keep stimulation within bounds. When you limit the draw on your energy pie, you will have more stamina when emotional modulation occurs.

What About My Life?

Good question. Do you get to have a life? Certainly, but differently. Your life right now is focused on healing your brain. But what about next week, next month, and next year? What then?

Will I have to start over? Who will I be when I get well? I pondered this constantly, reflecting upon the options. Here's what the journal looked like one day.

JOURNAL ENTRY NOVEMBER 17, 1992

For the last two weeks I've been flooding myself with catalogues to chiropractic schools and acupuncture schools. Do I go back to college for three years of science prerequisites, then four years of chiropractic school, and live in Iowa or Texas or Oregon, taking on a $200K loan to pull it off? Not to mention being 50 when I graduate?

Or go to acupuncture school in Denver or Boulder, a three-year proposition, $15,000, and screen out most of my weddings while I keep working full time and add an extra 30 hours per week to my work life?

Who am I kidding? Where do the three books fit in? I haven't turned on my Macintosh computer yet and the Nordic Track sits silently most evenings. Simple discipline has not returned. Or is there still no room in my head for these activities?

Or is this all about respect? For myself and for others. If I limp along in my practice (why do I see it as limping?), am I loving myself the most? Will Dan love me if I don't go back to school? Will I love myself if I don't change my livelihood? Is impatience rearing its ugly head? Will weddings keep me intellectually satisfied? Will writing keep me financially encouraged? What do I love the most and how do I know? Is time truly a factor here? Do I have to die with all my bills paid? If money were not the issue, which path would I choose?

Would I live elsewhere, love someone new, change jobs, change personalities, keep skiing, keep volunteering, get a dog?

Summary

Starting over may be your outcome. Your lifestyle will incur change as your brain heals. Changes great and small await you. See the chapter "New Abilities and New Skills" for more insights and options.

4

For Family Members

Every member of your family must read this chapter. That's an order. Someone in your family has been injured in a way that is different from a broken leg or an infectious disease. Brain injuries can be complicated and may involve soft tissue damage and physical pain. Recovery time may take months or a few years, or the injuries may remain only partially resolved.

Your family member may sustain changes in cognitive ability, (i.e., thinking skills), personality, and memory. These changes may be temporary, partially permanent or permanent. They may affect your relationship with your loved one.

The stress for you may be just as overwhelming as it is for your injured loved one. This chapter "For Family Members" discusses the stresses, the anger and frustration, the financial strain, the effects on family dynamics, and the solutions to help you cope with this change in the family lifestyle. Make no mistake. Your family lifestyle has changed. No, you weren't consulted.

What Happened?

Someone in your family has been injured in a way that may not appear obvious to you. His injury may make you feel uncomfortable, abandoned, helpless, unloved, ignored, enslaved, depressed, angry, vulnerable, less important to the family, overworked, or numb.

If that person is your child, your feeling of helplessness will likely increase, and frustration will compound the issue. Your child's behavior may be different.

You will need to relearn this child in order to take care of her. You may have to take back responsibilities that your child had assumed before the injury. You may lose some of your well-earned independence.

If that person is your spouse, anger about abandonment of the relationship may be your concern. Your marriage as you know it, with its sharing of burdens as well as loving affections, may be gone or put on hold. You may acquire added financial and household responsibilities that will put you close to the edge. It is all very painful and exhausting and demands an extra measure of valiant courage and character.

Your loved one may be temporarily or permanently changed in any number of ways. Recovery and return of function may take months or several years or may shift incrementally for an undetermined period of time. Everything from memory to social functioning to personality traits to professional capacity may (but does not have to) shift.

You may not like what you see. You may be frightened, angry, distressed, stressed, and emotionally challenged in ways you never pictured for your life. Your life, and the life of your loved one and your other family members, now requires an extra dose of courage and love.

You may experience a number of societal expectations about your role as caretaker. During this time, you may not feel it is appropriate to take care of yourself. However, if you are not taking care of yourself or accepting help and support from others, you won't be in a strong, healthy, balanced position to take care of your loved one.

The Injured Person First Comes Home

When the head-injured person first comes home (usually from the doctor or the hospital), it is a happy family event for all. It is also, however, just the beginning of the recovery process. The obvious physical injuries (bruises, fractures) are soon healed. The head injury, which we all hope will heal in a few months, can in reality take years. As the months pass, the healing benchmarks become more subtle. Your loved one starts to look "normal."

Fatigue will be a major factor. Your loved one may have only a few strong hours a day for thinking, moving about, and attending medical appointments and therapy. Mornings are best for therapy appointments or any critical planning. By afternoon, he can be "on the couch" for the remainder of the day and evening.

When friends drop by to celebrate the return of your family member, usually it's most convenient for them to come in the evening, just when the brain-injured person is at his lowest energy levels. Consider inviting friends over on the weekend, in the morning. Limit the event to half an hour at first. Gauge visitors' time to your loved one's energy. Be firm and keep visitation boundaries.

"The Patient"

In the rush to care and serve your loved one, the pressures can be overwhelming. Often, references to the head-injured person start to slip into the third person, speaking above her, around her, about her. You may unintentionally begin to speak down to her or omit her from conversations concerning her, even in the room in front of her!

Your injured family member wants to be treated like a present person whose life is repairing and moving forward. Review your state of mind, and observe your need for control, possible caretaking issues you bring to the relationship, and possible unnecessary sacrifice or martyr mentality.

Your loved one needs you. In a balanced, peaceful way.

Stress

Each individual experiences stress differently. Self knowledge is important here so that you can monitor your stress levels during this experience. Almost everything—including indigestion, insomnia, allergies, hair loss, heart palpitations, hemorrhoids, panic attacks, edginess, mood swings, and zits—can be traced back to stress. Know how you react so that you can be gentle with yourself and care for your needs accordingly.

Research suggests that it may take up to six months after an initial injury of your loved one for her symptoms to fully develop. You will need to get out for some fun, get some space from your loved one occasionally, and maintain your personal life routine as much as possible. Enhance your nutrition and exercise regimens.

Anger

No, you did not invite this event into your life. Anger can easily build up around the situation in which you find yourself. Anger can also build up and be directed toward your loved one or can be displaced and taken out on others. Psychotherapy is a good idea for the whole family. It will allow more open lines of communication, reduce stressors, and improve familial cooperation. Family counseling will provide you with information that furthers your understanding of your situation. Brain injury support-based psychotherapy offers you constructive alternatives for your family life.

Frustration

It can really drive you crazy when you are used to a certain level of cognitive performance from your loved one and he cannot live up to it or can't do it consistently anymore. The family has to slow down to the speed of the slowest member. If that member used to be the leader, this will confuse the relationships and alter family dynamics and the chain of command.

You may have to repeat yourself often. You may be dealing with a depressed person exhibiting mood swings and low energy. You may have to come home from work and still do everything in the house. Resentment is likely to creep in if your perception of this piece is out of balance. It's okay to ask for help from friends. Yes, even with the dishes. People really want to help you. Give them something to do.

You Need Support

The same ideas expressed in the chapter "Support Systems" also apply to you. If life becomes too overwhelming, you can and must get help. Your lifestyle will usually not improve without a helping hand. Embarrassing? Sure, everyone likes to think she can handle cooking, cleaning, shopping, and clutter. Relax. We've all been there at some time. Give yourself the gift of support.

Financial Strain

If your loved one was a financial participant, or if your insurance company is falling short on promised benefits, or both, financial strain is likely. Each family solves financial problems in a unique way. A family meeting to discuss the options and necessary adjustments is in order. Involve everyone, since the lifestyle of the group is on the table.

You will likely need to pull in the financial belt on your lifestyle and shift into frugal mode. Without knowledge of the duration of your loved one's condition, financial matters must be in your full control during this time. A financial planner or your attorney can be helpful. Consult your local bookstore for guidance on living at your new means.

Lifestyle Changes

Your lifestyle will change. You have someone at home for whom you must provide care, you have to go to work, you have extra chores when you return home. Your loved one may be sleeping most of the time and have no interest or motivation to pursue fun. Vacations will usually be exhausting. Movies are often too loud, violent, and crowded. The grocery store is too bright, loud, overstimulating, and intimidating. Restaurants can be claustrophobic, overwhelming, and too noisy.

You may need to seek recreation away from your loved one, since she really may not be up to the task. She may not have the energy to have fun. All of her energy is being spent healing her brain.

Furthermore, your loved one may not be able to participate in usual family activities. Reentry into the world of play will take time. For instance, it took me six months before I could ski again. It took a year before I would even consider riding my bike. It took two years before I could rock climb. It took two years before I went on a car trip by myself. Whatever your recreations, returning to them takes time. You certainly will require fun before then. Plan accordingly. You may be pleasantly surprised to discover that some hospitality and recreation establishments will accommodate your loved one's special needs. Just ask! (It's good business practice to accommodate customers!)

Your loved one will also begin to make new friends. As the previous cadre of pals shakes out (some will remain friends, others will drift away for a variety of reasons), new people will come into the circle. It is important to allow new relationships to build. Give your loved one the space to explore new friends and new interests.

The Emotional Rollercoaster

Your loved one will likely show signs of depression. Mood swings are common and not intentional. Irrational behavior, inconsolable crying, flashes of anger, perhaps physical outbursts, and long moments of staring off into space are a few of the general symptoms associated with the mood changes accompanying brain dysfunction. Your loved one would do anything to avoid feeling and acting as he does. He is powerless to control the hormonal or biochemical shifts the brain generates. To assist the doctors, record these episodes in a journal.

There are constructive ways in which to structure the environment of your loved one so that he will have as much energy as possible to devote to emotional modulation. Strategize the day. Avoid putting your loved one in a position where he is likely to tire quickly or become overstimulated. Planning can spare a great deal of exhaustion for him and ultimately for you. Ask him what over stimulates or tires him. The answers will surprise and enlighten you. Your accommodation and understanding will ease the experience.

Your Loved One Does Not Look the Least Bit Sick

There is little, if any, external evidence that a brain injury has taken place. No blood; no harm done. We associate sickness with casts, crutches, scars, blood, green skin, barfing, limps, slouching, facial changes, and weird smells. When the person staring off into space on the couch looks fine, it is difficult to generate a sympathetic response. You are used to responding to an external clue of injury.

Aside from lethargy, a short attention span, and altered sleeping habits, this person looks more than capable of doing laundry, vacuuming, or at least watering the plants sometime during the day. Quite honestly, she may not be capable of it, at least initially.

There were days when my most active task was walking outside to collect the mail. There were mornings when I had only enough energy to either pour cereal into a bowl for breakfast *or* eat the cereal in the bowl. But not both.

Your loved one is definitely injured and may take several years to recover all that she is capable of recovering. This will vary from person to person, and from year to year. The most obvious improvements usually take place in the first two years. Subtle improvements may continue for the rest of your loved one's life.

The Brain: A Simple Discussion

The brain is the central control mechanism for all functions in the body. Each part of the brain has its own jobs to perform, and the parts of the brain are interconnected and interdependent (see the figure below). When a portion of the brain is bruised, traumatized or damaged, the job it performs may be reduced in efficiency or eliminated, either temporarily or permanently.

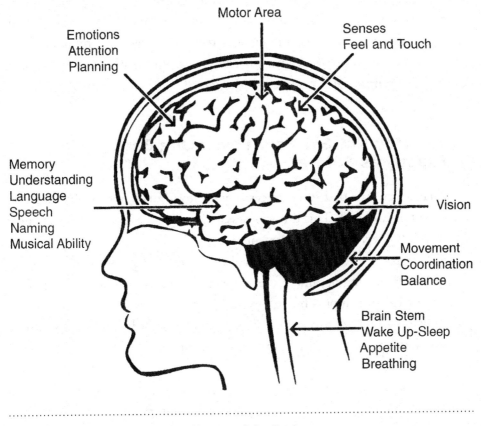

Diagram of the Brain

Learn all you can about the brain. Ask your healthcare provider for references to research books, articles, and web sites on brain function. Not at the rocket-science level, but at the lay level. Books and magazine articles will introduce you to the incredible world of the human brain. A healthy overview of information will serve you well.

Learn about the cognitive (thinking), physical, and emotional tasks the brain performs. Explore and discover the hormones, chemicals, and other communications that the brain monitors and controls. You will be amazed, fascinated, and impressed by what you learn. The human brain performs countless intricate jobs. For your loved one, some functions are currently performing less efficiently.

Pay attention to anatomy vocabulary. With the use of the diagrams you find, visualize the mechanism of injury for your loved one. Note the general areas that may have been impacted in the injury. This information will assist you now in comprehending the injury and will serve you later in understanding and translating legal, medical, and insurance terms. The challenge ahead may require you to understand fully all of this and more.

So, there is homework. As usual, it pays off in the long run. Family members who can speak and understand technical jargon get more and better answers to their questions and more respect from the healthcare, legal and insurance communities. Knowledge is power.

You May Not Get Your Loved One Back Exactly as Before

Chances are fair that some pieces of your loved one's personality, however small, will be different. This is not necessarily a negative aspect. Some changes can be productive, creative, and encouraging.

Although my eyesight was dimmed a bit and I required a stronger prescription, my hearing became more acute and sensitive. I now prefer Mozart, whereas Led Zeppelin puts me in physical pain.

I can now spell words backwards as well as forwards. Hardly a skill one puts on a resume, just a silly example of new talents available to the healing person.

Your loved one may change professions. If a near-death experience was a part of the injury, thoughts on death and spirituality may shift as well. One thing is certain. Life changes us, however subtly, every day. Your loved one will never be exactly the same. However, he may develop a new perspective on life that includes a more profound appreciation of life and loved ones like you.

The Energy Pie and You

Normally, healthy people have a store of energy to call upon in daily life and during times of emergency or stress. People who have been brain injured lose their extra reserve of energy and have nothing to call upon when the normal supply is exhausted. This can explain activity one minute and staring off into space the next.

Please refer to the chapter "Stamina, Fatigue, and Energy" for a more comprehensive overview of the energy-pie phenomenon. Your loved one has limited energy—physical, emotional, mental—and it is vital to understand that. What looks like idleness to you may be simply a lack of energy reserve.

You May Get Someone Even More Special

Your loved one may be more sensitive, loving, unconditional, and giving than before. That's not so bad. Outcomes can be most positive, so look for the positive ones. Grieve for the loss of your former relationship, but keep an open mind and an open heart about the new relationship that is unfolding. You may find yourself falling in love all over again.

Family Dynamics

The power shift that takes place in a family when one member suddenly requires more attention and resources is important to note. It is difficult to pay close attention to the needs of all family members when you feel you must remain focused on your injured loved one. A family therapist may be most valuable in assisting your family to create strong, productive, and supportive lines of communication. Some insurance companies will pay for family therapy sessions. Get professional advice on family dynamics. Visit your local brain-injury support group.

Unconditional Love

Long-term recovery from a brain injury takes courage, patience, and understanding. Everyone needs courage for the loved one to triumph over her injuries. New heights in unconditional love are reached as each family member rises to the challenge. Undeniable growth will take place for the family dedicated to staying together and making this work. It is an ultimate challenge of love and relationship. The effort is worth it. Each family member will emerge with a matured level of love, trust, and compassion for themselves, for each other, and for the injured member.

Brain injury isn't for slackers, and neither is family love. This experience can take you to the edge of your patience, tear you apart, and then make you stronger. Life is full of unanticipated experiences. Personal strength comes from living and loving beyond expectation into reality.

Home Safety Checklist

On a more practical level, the following suggestions, though obviously common sense, are prudently reviewed and may be critical when there is a brain-injured person in the house. Frequently, your loved one may have impaired vision or hearing. Balance may not be secure, and she may have difficulty remembering what was done or started five minutes ago. Your loved one may not be able to perceive how she has recently changed. Double check your home to be sure you are doing your best to avoid an unnecessary household mishap or injury.

- ○ Check for safely located electrical cords. Run them along baseboards, not under carpeting. No frayed or cracked cords. All cords must be properly grounded, and all extension cords must be adequate for their intended use.

- ○ Post all emergency numbers by each phone. Add pen and paper to each location.

- ○ Check smoke alarms and carbon monoxide alarms for proper working order.

- ○ Monitor kitchen activities, especially cooking. Short-term memory loss contributes to leaving pots on the stove unattended. The same applies for power tools and equipment in the garage. Supervision or follow-up are advised.

- ○ Check the location and operation of space heaters. Monitor wood-burning stoves.

- ○ Anchor rugs and carpets with nonskid backings. Keep all walkways clear and clean.

- ○ Adjust your hot water heater to 120 degrees or lower. Install nonskid strips on the bathtub or shower floor.

- ○ Test all hand railings for stability.

- ○ Install a nightlight in or near the bedroom of the loved one. Provide a stable lamp near the bed. Monitor electric blanket use, as the brain-injured person may not be able to accurately sense heat.

Summary

So, here are some positive suggestions. Seek family therapy that centers on family dynamics and communication with a professional trained in brain dysfunction. Take care of your needs. Get outside help. Ask for support. Read the rest of this book so that you will understand your loved one's experience.

Consult an attorney if your insurance company tries to settle early or isn't following through with appropriate benefits. Work with all the identified healthcare professionals and journal your meetings and conversations each time. Create a file and a journal of all contacts with medical, legal, and insurance people. If you keep track from the beginning, when and if all these folks decide to argue, it won't make you quite as crazy. Document everything.

Get a massage for yourself on a regular basis. Self care is most important for you. A little bit of sanity will go a long way during the stressful times. Keep love foremost in your mind. When sex is on your mind, read the chapter on "Sex" to better understand that aspect. Remain valiant, even though you, too, will have your awful days. Return to your still point of courage and resourcefulness. Know that you will succeed. Keep your eye on the prize.

5

Support Systems

Attracting help and support when you first experience your accident may occur spontaneously. But, as the accident continues to take its toll, you may not look or act "sick." You may, in fact, appear just fine and function sufficiently to pass for "well."

Asking for support and help when it may not be an obvious need requires courage. Your own ego and self-esteem may challenge you. To get the help and support you need, you must examine yourself and your willingness to accept help.

This chapter discusses how to know what to ask for, how to focus on the job that needs doing, how to spread your requests around, and how to deal with the emotional issues of long-term need.

Your spouse or partner will be included in this chapter, as well as the chapter for family members. Brain injury can surely stress a relationship, and there are ways to work it out.

I Need Help

The first hurdle is to acknowledge that you need help, even if you don't look like you do—especially because you don't look like you do. You need help. It is precisely because you may not appear sick that you must ask for assistance. It is not necessarily obvious that you need continued help and support after the first few weeks of blatant or debilitating symptoms.

Yes, I Need Help

The details of life are exhausting, especially when incomplete sequencing, impaired executive function, and depression are your daily companions. Frustration contributes to the entire mess, and, before you know it, life seems completely out of control.

Once More with Feeling: I Need Help!

There are two kinds of help: real help and the busy work you give to others because you can't sort out your true needs. There are two stages of help: the help you need before you deal with the anger of your injury and the help you need after the anger begins to resolve itself.

Real Help and Busy Work

Real help deals with the daily details of living. Errand running, shopping, cleaning, doing laundry, vacuuming, doing dishes, plant watering, pet care, lawn care, opening and sorting the mail, cooking, and recycling are all daily routine activities. Ask for support in these areas. Be as clear as you can regarding when you need help and how much help you need. You are not completely ineffective, and you will benefit from performing tasks you realistically can do yourself. Just get help for the remaining tasks.

Busy work is more in the "can you get me a glass of water" category. Generally this shows that you either have no clue what needs to be done or you are unwilling to let go of the real work assignments. Hopefully you will recover from this stage before your plants die, your cat runs away, you have no clean underwear, or your neighbors turn you in to the city for having foot-high grass. Brain dysfunction is an explanation for your challenges, not an excuse for you to be waited on hand and foot.

Always Give Away the Jobs that Make You Cry

I found this rule very helpful. If I discovered that, by trying to do a job I instead melted into tears, it was my clue that I was overwhelmed. Give the jobs away that make you cry.

DECEMBER 23, 1992

> I cry a lot. A lot more than before. At little things, or things
> that seem little. Mostly things that remind me about my problem.
> Mostly ego-attached things. That throw it in my face and make
> me feel less . . . broken . . . no way out. In a deep hole, the edge
> of which reminds me of the "event horizon" of Steven Hawking's
> Black Hole. As if I lack the particle to bridge the event horizon;
> as if one could exit as easily as enter.
>
> I cry a lot. And this man stays, with warm and unconditional
> arms that wrap me in, cloak me in. Things will get better, he says.
> You are my jewel today. You will always be my jewel. He didn't
> know me before. He loves me blindly. When will I offer myself
> this gift?

Help Before Anger Work

The help you need before you work on your anger will be harder to ask for and more difficult to receive. All the "I shouldn't have tos" and "I used to be able tos" are still involved. This is a stage of your healing process, and it will pass once you work it out.

Help After Anger Work Begins

Once your healing process includes anger work (see the chapter "Anger"), you will gently discover that you are justified in asking for help. In fact, you are a help magnet, and assistance will come to you when and where you need it. Help is everywhere, for the asking. You are the perfect recipient of that help. Your support system will grow and flourish. People love helping you and seek you out to offer their assistance. (Close your eyes and let your heart hear these words.)

Control

Asking for help is all about control and self-esteem. It may seem that the brain injury has taken control of your life. Because you have always felt like you were in control, or always wanted control, the feeling of not having control makes for a fairly vulnerable and scary state of mind.

When your self-esteem is enmeshed with control issues and you are not in control, you also have a generally low opinion of yourself. This, with an overlay of biochemical depression, digs a very deep pit. People in pits have no control.

Asking for Help Is a Self-Esteem Issue

So, here we are again. Back to self-esteem. Frame your thinking so that asking for help validates how much you love and care for yourself. *Asking for help is a positive, productive, loving, caring, effective support for your healing process.* (Write that on a sticky note and put it on the bathroom mirror.)

Back at Work

You may not be able to do your whole job at first. You may have stamina for half days or three days a week. What about job sharing? It's trendy, smart, supportive, and productive and enhances your healing process. Your boss would rather have you part of the time than have to train someone else. You are valuable, and your boss will do whatever possible to keep your valuable services.

Job Coach

Job sharing is one way to support you at work. There are many other ways to return to work part time. Explore those options with your individual employer. Ask for a job coach or human resources person to assist you in staying at your job.

For the self-employed, hiring a part-time person to support your activities may offer you some relief. Ask for support from trustworthy associates. A good creative planning and management session may turn up options that work well.

Returning to School

Most universities are prepared to support your learning with special services. Head injury is a disability that qualifies for specific considerations.

You do need to ask for this support. Check with the student services office. Be prepared with a letter from your doctor or neuropsychologist demonstrating your documented needs.

Little things, like having a little extra time to take a test. Or to be able to take a test in a quiet room, without auditory (other students) or visual (bright lights or people moving about) distractions can make the difference.

Ask for study notes because you have a brain injury and may not be taking the greatest notes! What with having to pay attention to the lecture, write ideas down, and deal with bright lights, the jokesters sitting behind you, and the noise of shuffling chairs, your notes may not even capture the actual salient points of the topic. You may even qualify for a tutor. Take it. The school will support you to succeed.

You can make it through school with the support of those around you. The university wants you to succeed, and it has a system that supports your quest.

Support Systems: Case Manager

Consider choosing a case manager. This can be one of your present healthcare practitioners (preferably the one with the most holistic or all-encompassing view of your situation: someone who believes you and understands your condition) or an additional practitioner with a specialty in case management for brain injury. The special skills of the case manager will serve to track your therapies, keep the members of your healthcare team talking with each other and working together, monitoring for counterproductive treatments and affirming that you are improving. The case manager also makes sure your insurance company and all other nonmedical entities are cooperating with each other to your best advantage.

Support Systems: Friends

Allow your friends to help you. Receive their support. Create alliances that support your healing process. You will likely need a "walking buddy." You will need a "reading buddy" to go through your mail and keep your finances in order. A temporary bookkeeping service can organize and pay your bills and balance your checkbook.

I used to have breakfast buddies who would come over to my house on their way to work and eat breakfast with me. That ensured that I was out of bed, safely out of the shower, eating, and ensconced on the sofa at a civilized hour.

And what did I do in return? I thanked people as frequently as I could remember to. A hearty "thank you" can go a long way, especially when your helper knows it may be all you reasonably can do. Sometimes survivors can suck their helpers dry without considering what they can do to acknowledge their assistance. Sometimes, just being a friend back, listening, and offering your heart is the biggest gift you can give in return. Even with a brain injury, you can usually accomplish a modicum of appreciation and listening.

Support Systems: Community Services

Grocery stores will shop for you and deliver groceries. For a tip, some delivery people will put your groceries away! Video stores have delivery and online subscriptions. Errand-running services, housekeeping services, in-home cooking services, community bus systems for disabled people, and pet-walking services are available in many areas. Hire them.

If you have personal injury protection in your state from your auto insurance company, your policy may include a supportive services benefit. Your policy may provide per diem for support services that assist you in carrying on with your life. Ask your insurance agent or attorney about this.

Local high schools generally have a counselor who handles after-school student employment placement for chores. Ask about the fees.

Support Systems: Family Members

Life goes on in the family. Even in a loving family setting, you will look less and less sick. Your illness will wear not only on you, but also on those around you. Having a strong communication network in your family will assist you in expressing your needs and improve your opportunities for support and understanding.

When your family members live far away, they may have very little information about your condition, and even less opportunity to support you on a daily basis. It is important to tell the truth of your condition and not put on a happy face when they call. Being as truthful as possible will help to prevent your resenting them years later for not guessing how bad off you "really" were. (See the chapter "For Family Members.")

Support Systems: Spouse, Significant Partner

Relationship is life's hardest work. I believe a successful relationship is the greatest challenge we humans face. Strong positive relationships are the result of dedication, love, courage, and hard work.

A relationship is challenging enough without a brain injury thrown in to increase the degree of difficulty. Brain injury will test your relationship. It will also strain, push, vibrate, shake, twist, reshape, rehash, flashback, try, and unhinge your primary relationship.

Brain-injury recovery is hard work. You will likely be the passive partner for a while. Your energy only goes so far, and brain repair comes first. Your partner needs to know what to expect in the short and long term. Your partner has a right to know your condition and the projected length and general overview of the therapy required for recovery time.

Relationship Issue: You Might Not Be You Anymore

Your injury may have altered your personality in ways that are no longer attractive to your partner. Your injury may have changed your sex life (see the chapters "Sexual Response" and "Risk and Initiation"). The new you may not be able to fulfill the expectations, assumptions, and dreams of your partner. You might not be you anymore, in your partner's eyes. This can definitely put the relationship at risk.

What appears to be a life-altering injury may exceed your partner's strength of character. Your partner may not be able to cope and may choose to leave. You may feel abandoned. Self-blame may set in. Back to the self-esteem chapter!

Psychotherapy with a professional who understands brain dysfunction can be most valuable for retaining your relationship. Establishing or reestablishing lines of communication is vital to the survival of the relationship.

All couples have unique facets, angles, and personalities. We work out our agreements, renegotiating as we live with one another. With brain injury, all agreements are off. Reconstruction of your life as a couple, with possible long periods of limbo, is difficult at best.

FEBRUARY 11, 1993, PARTNERSHIP

This man I'm marrying (try planning a wedding in cognitive low gear!) is incredibly supportive. And although it is important to factor in that I did not know him before my fall (so he doesn't know what's missing or who I "used" to be and therefore he suffered no grief or loss), my projection and hope is that we would have weathered this experience in any case.

This may not be true for everyone. Relationships are all dynamically different, and the agreements/assumptions/agendas we express/repress come into play with long-term stress and long-term change/long-term alteration.

Life may not turn out as planned. If your partner holds you responsible for lost or stolen dreams, it could be very disappointing, even devastating, to the relationship. I know I'm different. Grit my teeth and repeat.

Humor Is Good

Keeping humor in the relationship is a balm of great use. We named my funny mistakes as coming from my "Lumbar Brain." (Limbic brain is the correct reference, for the anatomy challenged. Lumbar is low back or close to the buns area, as inferred by the error-plus-humor.) Laughing is good.

Going to the movies may be an answer to the problem, if the content will not overstimulate you and the crowd factor is within your comfort level. When your world is too full, and there is too much to do, a little entertainment may be the answer. Escape with humor and gentleness. Order pizza. Go for a walk. Just walk away from the tension for a while. A time-out is very good therapy.

Humor Entry

The trickster, represented by Coyote in Native American tradition, is a great way to shift blame. "Where are the car keys?" "Coyote hid them." Always looking for fun, or to play a prank, shifting blame to Coyote not only takes the pressure off you, it places blame squarely on the shoulders of the likely culprit. Once I surrender to Coyote trickstering, the car keys magically appear (in varying lengths of time).

Professional Help

Remember the value of the professionals in this process. Your physician, psychotherapist, neuropsychologist, or attorney may be your best support, depending upon your situation. The following article excerpt reveals an important point:

> The diagnosis of mild closed brain injury (or mild traumatic brain injury) has been elusive at best. It poses a problem for doctors, lawyers, insurance companies and most importantly, the patients themselves. It is frequently missed by physicians, psychologists, neuropsychological testing and traditional medical workups. In fact, in this author's experience, lawyers often diagnose it more accurately for their clients than many medical professionals.
>
> Patients suffer from depression, anxiety, confusion, sleep disturbances, irritability, mood lability, difficulty focusing, memory problems and inability to function in their previous employment. They feel little relief from the medical community, either because they are misdiagnosed, told it will go away with time or left feeling abandoned to suffer on their own with little effective treatment available.[2]

At the Doctor's Office

There is a special talent to speaking with your doctors about your situation. It is paramount that you are prepared for each meeting. Make a list of issues to discuss at each meeting with each practitioner. When you are prepared, the doctor will record your symptoms and complaints in your file. When you are not prepared, or just plain forget to bring up issues (because you have a brain injury and your memory is sketchy at best), you come off as a random, all-over-the-map complainer. When you have your little list, the doc has something on which to hang a diagnosis. And a solid diagnosis is the key to supported, long-term therapy.

Your doctor's medical notes are reviewed by the insurance company as decisions on payment for the services are considered. The doctor's notes are as informative as your report of your symptoms. Be clear, concise, and thorough. This is the true field upon which you prove your case. Consider reviewing your list with your spouse, family member, or good friend. This helps you record factors you may have overlooked or of which you may not be aware.

Make your list, maybe keep it on the fridge so, when you remember an issue, it is easy to jot down. On your calendar, next to your appointment notation, jot down to remember to take the list!

Keep Your Own Medical File

In this age of "medical privacy," the contents of your medical file, as it grows in each practitioner's office, may be less current than optimal. I highly recommend that you keep your own copy of your medical file with you at each appointment. You may have copies of tests, narratives, and reports in your file that your practitioner does not have. When you provide information, the appointments go more smoothly, and you get more efficient and informed care.

Make your file folder a bright color so it stands out to you visually and you can more easily remember to take it with you. Keep the information in chronologic order. *(Note to family members: If your loved one is currently unable to keep this file, it is paramount that you do it.)*

The Independent Medical Examination

If your health insurance or auto insurance company is involved with your recovery, the company will do its best to stay informed about your condition and your progress. Not all insurance companies are created equal. The IME, or independent medical examination, is a tool used by insurance companies to get a second opinion for their own information and evaluation of your status and progress.

Some insurance companies use their own doctors to evaluate you independently of your medical providers. For some companies, this exam is meant to ascertain your progress. For others, this exam is used to validate termination of benefits.

In recent history, the IME has been incorporated earlier and earlier in the recovery process, attempting to reduce the financial exposure of the insurance company. In the process, you, as the patient and insured, may feel discredited by the experience and even revictimized by it.

Your lawyer is trained to fight for your interests. Let your lawyer represent you to your insurance company. It is your task to make a psychological break with the insurance company so that you can focus on getting well.

It will be difficult, but do not take the IME or its subsequent results personally. Proceed with your healing process. Proceed with your medical treatments and regimens. Do not spend a drop of your valuable energy on anger. An anger-triggered relapse episode does not serve you. Use your energy wisely and continue your line of recovery work. (If, on the other hand, this strategy stuffs your emotions, then go for it. Get mad, express yourself, and then get over it. People are different. Select the path of action that works best for you.)

As your attorney well knows, the insurance companies usually end up paying in the end, even if the case drags on for years. That is why your lawyer works on a contingency basis.

It is the job of the insurance adjuster to save money for the insurance company. It is the lawyer's job to defend your right to your contractual benefits. It is your job to get well. Proceed with your therapy.

You can avoid many IMEs by insisting that all your healthcare professionals provide treatment plans, typed progress notes of every session, timely submission of your bills, and quick response to correspondence or phone calls from your adjuster. Generally, the insurance company wants data about your case. If it appears on their desk, there is generally less reason for an IME to learn what the company wants to know.

Summary

Support comes in many guises. Vacuuming, dishwashing, and plant watering are direct and obvious tasks. Job sharing, day-care sharing, and executive functions restore control, self – esteem, and a sense of productivity. Hugs and understanding and a good walk around the park support the soul.

Relationships are vital to support systems and to your optimal recovery rate. Support needs may last several years and may change in their requirements, category, and depth during that time. Ask for help. Ask for help. Then redefine what you need and ask for help again.

The copy below is the most current flyer I use when I teach a class for brain-injured people and their family members. It is a quick and useful summary. Please copy it and share it.

Building Your Support System

Brainlash, Maximize Your Recovery From Mild Brain Injury
Gail L. Denton, PhD

Who is a member of your support system?

Family members, friends, business associates, healthcare providers, your employer, your attorney, tax accountant, insurance company, gym, hobby association, your support group.

Why do you need a support system?

You have a brain injury and you need help navigating your return to wellness. You need support, guidance, professional expertise, therapy, medical attention, legal advice, and also time for leisure recreation and fun. You need someone to ensure that you are receiving what you need and when you need it. You need someone to track with you to ensure you are receiving the best possible recovery information and support. And, especially, you need someone to deal with your insurance company, your lawyer, and your healthcare professionals to certify that your progress is the best it can be.

Who leads your support system?

Some folks have willing family members who assist with this process. Others rely upon a case manager or healthcare provider who has agreed to serve the role of case manager. Stay mindful that, even if willing family members help out, professional advice is essential for proper management of your recovery and therapeutic supervision. It is vital not to 'burn out' your family members.

Remember, not all participants in your support system (insurance company, employer) may cooperate fully or understand your situation at all times during this process. Your support-system leader deals with these events, leaving the healing activities as your responsibility.

Your Medical Healthcare Providers

Primary care physician, additional physician specialists, physical therapist, occupational therapist, massage therapist, cranial sacral therapist, behavioral optometrist, dentist, chiropractor/osteopath, neuropsychologist, psychotherapist, acupuncturist, nutritionist, to name a few.

Your Complementary Healthcare Providers

Your gym or recreation center, your hobby groups, your vacation organizer, your support groups, your social groups, your spiritual groups. Exercise, music, social interchange, relationships, leisure time, and emotional support are all essential to your healing process.

Your Employer

As you return to work, or develop a new occupation, it is important to be honest with your employer about your stamina levels as you are working. Negotiate for conditions that support you. Breaks, walks, early/late arrival, early/late departure, part time. Include your support group leader at the meeting.

Your Attorney

If your recovery involves an attorney, make certain the attorney understands brain-injury issues and has experience and a successful track record helping people recover financially, both from the party responsible for your accident and the insurance company involved.

Your Tax Accountant

Consider consulting an accountant because health insurance costs, prescriptions, home nurse visits, copays, domestic help, uncovered medical expenses, and mileage to and from your appointments may allow you to deduct expenses. It's worth knowing about.

Insurance Company

Depending on the origin of your brain injury (car crash? fall?), your insurance company will have an opinion on the amount of coverage available to you. Your support team leader must understand and be willing to navigate and chronicle this series of transactions. Request an insurance company "manager" with whom you always communicate, to reduce misunderstandings and to maintain recourse with the insurance company. Stay mindful that appeals are always a choice. When you believe you are entitled to benefits, continue to pursue those benefits regardless of initial denials by claims workers. Remember, rarely are the claims managers answering the phones. Only deal with true decision makers.

Your Pre-existing Condition

No one experiences a brain injury with a "clean slate" of health. We all have "pre-existing" conditions of one sort or another. It may be so routine that you don't realize it at first. Elevated blood pressure, menopause, seasonal allergies, excess weight, physical inactivity, a bum knee, or indigestion. Remember that your brain injury can sway these sorts of pre-existing conditions. Pay attention to these issues as well.

Hot Tips for Your Support System Leader

Gain the cooperation of the various healthcare providers. The treatment plan goal is to have no more than two appointments in any one day, preferably back to back. Minimize driving and maximize benefit. The goal is to have no more than three days a week for appointments. (Integration time for the received therapies is very important.) Appointments on Monday, Wednesday, Friday is an idea of a good place to start. See what works for optimal results.

When combining appointments, book the "active appointment" first and the "passive appointment" second. Book the appointments in order of benefit. For instance, book the massage before the chiropractor, book the exercise before the acupuncturist, book the dentist before the massage. Don't book two "talking" appointments back to back (example: occupational therapy, then psychotherapy) as that is exhausting. And don't book two "painful" appointments back to back. Revisit the treatment plan every two weeks.

Experimentation with the order of things is vital to learn what is working for the recovery plan. Observe what is improving the relative health and stamina. As time passes, the order of therapies may change, and also the kinds of therapy will change. The ultimate goal is to begin exchanging medical and therapeutic appointments with exercise and activity appointments.

Keeping a brain-injured person actively exercising is very important. Flexibility, stamina, and fresh air are vital ingredients in the recovery process. Exercise is a healthcare appointment.

(Copyright 2006 by Gail L. Denton.)

6

Work

Going back to work or school (or staying at work or in school) following a mild brain injury is an incredible challenge. Your ability to focus, act in a professional manner, study, learn, and even maintain your energy throughout the day are major concerns.

This chapter addresses the issues surrounding your ability to carry on your vocation or livelihood and offers suggestions for adapting your old world to the new you.

FEBRUARY 7, 1992

You look just fine to the external world.

Going Back to Work

Returning to work may not be a choice for you. Most of us must work in order to provide for ourselves. The extent of your injuries may prevent you from working at all. If so, how will you evaluate when you can return to work, and under what conditions?

It is not uncommon for people to report adaptive problems upon returning to work, school, or their previous activity level. Your life activity level will be different. You may not be as active or as able to activate yourself to "do" life.

You may not have the stamina to complete a day or a week of work. Even half a day, once or twice a week, may be the limit of your energy.

You may experience slow or fuzzy thinking, or you may find you are less efficient or productive than you remember.

Pace yourself. Do not expect your performance to be at the same level as before your accident. You may need help adjusting to the cognitive, emotional, and behavior changes you will experience when you return to work.

Workplace Advocate

When you return to work, you will look fine. There will be no obvious signs of your injury. No cane, crutch, cast, or bandage—nothing that looks remotely like illness to the untrained colleague. However, chances are you will be a mess inside. You will be tired, overwhelmed, overstimulated, slow to sort tasks and organize your day, and quick to rest. Your work may be less accurate than you expect of yourself. Your attention span may be shorter, and you could be prone to staring off into space. Paying attention at a meeting may be close to impossible.

You need a *workplace advocate.*

A workplace advocate will be helpful in interpreting your needs to your employer. Ask for such a person so that you will be perceived as receiving help. In a smaller company, the advocate may be the employer. In a larger organization, consult with the human resources department and request such a person. You may also wish to privately consult with a vocational rehabilitation specialist. Some insurance companies include this healthcare provider in their policies.

Your employer should be advised of the nature of your deficits and assist when possible in restructuring your job so that you will be more successful at it. Working with your environment so that you will succeed, adjusting your hours to maximize your abilities while nurturing your healing process, and being sensitive to changes in your needs are vital to your success and your employer's satisfaction. You may even need a leave of absence until you can return to work part time.

You may be able to return to work with few or no workplace accommodations, except perhaps for more frequent and longer breaks in the day. You may also discover that, when you present your needs for accommodation to your employer, you may be forced out of your job. Work with your employer and workplace advocate, and keep your attorney close by.

The workplace advocate will also help to offer you support as you re-enter the workforce. She may help you obtain the correct perspective regarding your return, offering you encouragement when a bad brain day hits. She may remind you that you are not sloughing off but, in fact, rehabilitating and recovering from a serious injury. Resist the urge to allow your own ego to get in the way of recovery, especially at work. Our culture wraps identity with occupation. ***You are not your job.*** You are a healing person, who offers gentle, caring compassion to yourself as you return to work.

MARCH 26, 1992: WHO AM I AT WORK?

> The old me seems gone. At least that's the report from my business partners who remember the fire in my eye and the gazillion ideas per minute that could pour forth on any given topic. They say my creativity is gone. The hard, clear brain factory of options. In its place, a more timid, soft, less committed energy has appeared, so they say.
>
> And that certainly isn't the old me. No it isn't. And I miss that staccato firebrand part of me that latched on and never let go until reality was at hand. I mourn the loss, however temporary.
>
> Parts of me are returning. Parts not. Yet other aspects are surfacing. (For the first time? As compensating balance? Were they always there, waiting a chance through the onslaught of louder, more outwardly powerful notions?) Aspects more quiet, subtle, peaceful perhaps.

The First Week Back

Questions may flood the mind on those first weeks back at work. Questions of self-doubt are at the top of the list. Can I still do my job? Do I want to continue in this profession? Can I think clearly enough right now to even ask those kinds of questions? Does my brain work well enough to try something new at this time? You may want to give yourself some time before tackling these premature queries.

APRIL 1, 1992

> It seems the intuition is back, and with it a renewed sense of purpose and ability to remain in my profession, at least for the time being.

Ever since the accident I have been convinced that my brain wouldn't somehow allow me to continue. That I have to find something else to do.

Professional Liability

There are certain professions, of course, that carry a serious level of professional liability with them. Confidentiality, professional secrets, customer concerns, research, medicine, technical performance, and others require levels of proficiency that must be maintained for credibility and liability. It is reasonable to ask oneself if the required level of proficiency is present. Are you performing adequately for yourself, the company, and the client?

Can my job responsibilities be temporarily adjusted, rescheduled, altered, changed or proctored to ensure quality in the workplace? Can I enroll a supportive supervisor to check my details? Must I ask myself if I can honestly perform what is expected of me right now? Is my job too difficult or overwhelming at the moment? Remember, it is important to be honest. It is also important to be gentle with yourself. Expecting perfection may be expecting too much.

A vascular surgeon may want to take more time off. A production manager may just need a few naps and a two-hour lunch. Ask for help and support in evaluating this situation.

Work Hardening

After a person has been away from the workplace for a while, getting back into the groove can be stressful. Getting up early, getting out the door, being on time, working all day, and returning home at the end of the day are all skills gained and honed over years of experience. Your stamina may not be up to the total task 100% when you return to work.

Working your way back to full employment gradually may be a reasonable alternative. Can you work part time or have flex time? What would work for you? What would work for your employer? Decisions that are focused on conserving energy and enhancing your attention span have a better chance of succeeding. A vocational rehabilitation specialist can help evaluate these issues. Together you can develop a "work-hardening" or stamina-increasing program of rehabilitation tailored to your needs. Include driving as a part of your daily-effort tally. Drive to avoid rush hours. Consider shorter workdays as full days when the drive time is included in the equation.

Money

Can I live on the adjusted salary that part-time employment provides? How well can I support myself and heal, too? Will my life crash around me if I cannot work? Will I crash if I return to work too soon?

Can I produce at 50% of normal? Can I adjust my lifestyle to accommodate my healing process? If I produce at 85% of normal proficiency, will anyone at work even notice? Am I the only one who knows I'm half a sandwich shy of a brown bag lunch?

Making money is a very challenging issue when brain injury is a factor. As hard as it may seem, you may find yourself unable to work and in need of financial assistance. Ask your family or friends for support.

You may have to rely on savings or cash in investments, get a second mortgage on your home, live on credit cards or sell belongings. Hopefully, your situation will not take you that far. If it does, consult an adviser before making financial decisions that you may not be able to fully understand. Life will go on. Lifestyle changes may alter your life for a while.

Self-Respect

Our society defines us by our work-related roles. We have a conscious identity with what we produce. When what we do is taken away, personal identity goes with it. The questions of self-doubt creep in and self-examination begins. Do I have self-respect at work with this injury?

There is a shred of wrong-headedness about this line of questioning. Consider, for a moment, that ***you are not your job.*** If you are not your job, then, if you have a new job (like getting well) or no job, then you are still a person with value to yourself and your community.

This is a good place to begin. ***You are not your job.***

Now, consider applying work to your life when it is healthy to do so. Consider removing work from your life when it is unhealthy. Would you make different choices about your vocation if health were your main consideration?

Of course, none of this makes the mortgage any smaller. It does, however, give you more mental breathing room in which to make healthy, balanced choices for yourself. How you structure your healing process now will pay dividends and interest in the years ahead.

Getting Dressed for Work

The value of sequencing was never more clear to me than when I tried to dress for work. In the workplace, dress code matters. Appropriate dress for your rank, position, or activity is extremely important.

For instance, as a psychotherapist in private practice, it is important for me to dress in a calm, conservative, and nonprovocative manner. Revealing blouses, tight or short skirts, cleavage, hot make-up, trendy outfits, flashy hair, or fashion-statement accessories are not conducive to the work environment. Making an uninhibited fashion choice could send a patient into orbit for any number of reasons. Dressing appropriately for me was more than important. It was a matter of ethics in the care of my patients.

JANUARY 25, 1993

> Getting dressed. Preparing to leave the house. Normal enough tasks. But if your brain isn't ready, you'll wear a black bra under a pink blouse or gold earrings and a silver necklace, forget to brush your teeth or hair, and arrive at work with slippers on and your glasses on the dining room table. For the longest time, I couldn't put my make-up on because I couldn't remember how. What colors went where. So I just quit wearing it for a while, so I wouldn't stare at myself in the mirror every morning.
>
> Most of my wardrobe has gone untouched. Safety in repetition. Certain outfits, certain earrings, certain shoes. Hang the once-a-week rule. Safe, boring outfits are the new order of the day.

Pacing

Working slowly can be important at first. Allowing your brain to get used to the pace of work will allow it to work longer and more effectively.

Fuzzy thinking can happen when the pace is too fast and all the brain parts cannot keep the pace.

Pacing is crucial. If you forget to pace yourself, the brain will shut down and you will end up losing more time in the long run. You cannot push the river. Your brain will be telling you how fast and for how long. You are only in charge of how often you overload the system. Pay attention and adopt pacing as a strategy.

IF NOT, THIS IS A LIKELY SCENARIO: MARCH 21, 1992

Going back to work was another matter. Reading and writing patient charts was not an option, it was a legal responsibility.

Months later, the blurring in my eyes comes back. Sometimes when I've overexerted, sometimes not. Stress is a factor, fatigue, mental exhaustion.

I've come to accept and even push through the fuzzy times, like now. My brain is working OK. I'm not in command of the greatest choice in words. There are several things I'm supposed to read this weekend, and a piece of a baby quilt I agreed to needlepoint. Fat chance. The reading is fuzzy, easier if held at arm's length. Sewing will have to wait until the tiny little threads can be seen and appreciated for their fine, delicate nature.

Mostly I feel caught, handicapped, held up, robbed, relieved of connection. Dead in the water.

Occupational Therapy

You can learn more about the process of work hardening and pacing with the help of an occupational therapist or vocational rehabilitation specialist familiar with the issues of mild brain injury. Many insurance policies cover this.

Preventive Work Reintegration

This is like defensive driving. When re-entering the workplace, operate in your own best interest. Document what you do, when you do it, and why you do it. Your return to work may not be smooth. You may have to file a complaint with the EEOC (Equal Employment Opportunity Commission) to keep your job. Whatever you do, don't quit. Make them fire you. Document, document, document!

Summary

Return to work as a healthy part of your healing process, but be honest with yourself about your level of ability. Proceed slowly and confidently. Ask for a workplace advocate. Taper your re-entry to match your energy level. Re-evaluate frequently, giving yourself the benefit of alternative routes, should your original path prove too taxing. Be gentle with yourself.

7

Driving

Your car is a very powerful machine. It is capable of getting you where you want to go. It is freedom. It is also a dangerous vehicle, which only does what you tell it to do. When the complicated functions of operating a motor vehicle are overwhelming, confusing, or exhausting, you are not ready to drive your car. Returning you to your car is a brutal error in your rehabilitation. The healthcare community is dropping the ball therapeutically. Your perception, motor skills, information integration, visual perceptual time frame, and response time are impaired. If you are driving without comment from your recovery support team, it is tantamount to inviting you to compound your life with yet another accident. Presently, 60%+ of brain-injured people re-injure themselves, often multiple times. What are we thinking?

This chapter points out the complicated processes necessary to drive safely. Refrain from driving until you can safely operate your vehicle. Consider taking driving school as a way to identify your skill level.

Your Eyes

With brain injury, there can be a time distortion between what your eyes see, when that information registers in the brain, and when your muscles can react to the information. Because of this issue, driving can be a dangerous enterprise. This skill is called "visual perceptual speed" and is vital to driving safely.

Your eyes team up to perceive the world. If they are not working well together, you will not see the world accurately, you will become visually fatigued, or both. A behavioral optometrist is a vital addition to your healthcare professional team. Get evaluated. Further explanation of the role your eyes play in driving is found in the chapter "Vision."

Driving

A great number of skills are involved in driving a car: cognitive abilities, hand-eye coordination, quick reaction time, self-correction, full attention, rational and logical thinking, self-regulation, and discernment are a few of the basic requirements for driving. Why, then, is driving not a skill assessed and rehabilitated, especially in the face of the obvious consequences: another accident.

Driving while recovering from a brain injury may tax your energy stores, making you exhausted, anxious, or confused. It may be difficult for you to focus your mind on the driving itself. Your depth perception may falter; decisions won't come quickly enough.

Driving requires, among other things, your ability to

- Make quick decisions
- Filter out traffic noise
- Filter out traffic speed
- Filter out traffic pressure
- Perceive and react to traffic signs and signals
- Filter out anxiety
- Operate a vehicle
- Remember where you are going
- Remember where you are at present
- Sequence events
- Remember how to drive the car in snow, ice, rain, and wind
- Follow a map

○   Relax if you get lost

○   Remember where you parked the car

○   Remember to add gas, oil, tires, water, antifreeze, and windshield liquid

○   Keep five dollars in the car just for gas

In traffic, there are numerous distractions such as noise, the radio, the activity of passengers in the car, bad weather, unsafe drivers, and rush-hour traffic. In addition, you may have episodes of defocusing your eyes. An energy drain may occur while you are driving, and your eyes or brain may slow or shut down for brief periods of time. You may focus on objects too long. Then, when you refocus, objects may be closer than you anticipated. You may even find yourself tailgating. Has society or your self-image pushed you behind the wheel too soon?

It is all too common that a brain-injured person finds herself in a mild fender bender due to visual decompensation. The figures are a staggering 60%+ for subsequent re-injury, and, frequently, that includes third, fourth, and fifth additional accidents. Prevent this. Wait to drive until you are ready. Really ready. Take driving school, like Master Drive. They specialize in driving training for brain-injured people.

Stress

You may discover that the overall stress of driving a car is too much for you. If you cannot drive at least 25 MPH without anxiety, you are not ready to drive, with or without a coach. For your own safety, rely on your support system for transportation until you are more fully capable. Our mobile society links success with transportation and issues of independence, freedom, and personal identity. If you can't drive, you perceive yourself as "handicapped." This social stigma pressures many recovering people to drive before they are ready. Climbing back behind the wheel is not necessarily a sign of recovery.

In the meantime, you can be treated for the problem with psychotherapy, behavioral optometry, cognitive retraining, and a new technique called eye movement desensitization reprocessing (EMDR). This therapy is remarkable in its simplicity and effectiveness. Causing no pain or discomfort and similar to hypnotherapy in its effectiveness, EMDR is a handy therapy tool. Many psychotherapists are trained in this technique, especially those versed in brain dysfunction therapies. (Beware the "weekend seminar" trained. Look for stronger qualifications.)

Get a Map

No matter how "easy" the directions sound, draw yourself a map to your destination and include landmarks and written directions with the address and phone number. When short-term memory and sequencing skills are impaired, a little map will get you where you need to go. It may even be helpful to have a map to your own home in the car. I drove myself to my old house numerous times and had to really think about how to get home.

Other People's Maps

Always ask questions about any map given to you. Most maps include assumptions (which will always get you in trouble), so find out distances and ask for landmarks that mean something to *you*. Include the name, address, and phone number of the destination on the map. Also include "if you have gone too far" landmarks as well. For this situation and many more, consider purchasing a cellular phone and a map of your town.

Being Overwhelmed

Sensory overload is certainly possible while driving. It is always your option to pull over and rest. When you feel tired, do not continue to drive. You could easily hurt yourself and others. Or end up having to converse with a police officer. You may not get a ticket, but you will have been driving while impaired. And you know it.

Am I Ready To Drive?

Evaluations that determine your driving readiness are available through your optometrist, neuro-ophthalmologist, cognitive rehabilitation specialist, driving school, or neuropsychologist. Tests can help determine if you have recovered sufficiently to drive. Other feedback, from passengers in your car or other motorists or law enforcement, can be a clear indication of readiness. If your first accident was in a car, the urge to get back on the horse can override logic. Until you heal, every time you get behind the wheel you relive the crash. This emotional overlay only compounds a task you are ill prepared to perform. Avoid subsequent injury. Add driver training to your rehab schedule.

Handy Hint for Parking the Car

Attach a red ball or colorful ribbon to the radio antenna of your car. I attach a ribbon to my ski rack. When you are looking for your car in a parking lot, the extra device will help you find your car (or the car of another brain-injured person with a ski rack, but I digress). Choose a device that will work best for you. When you park in a garage or at the airport, carry a sticky note to record your location. The note will guide you back to your car.

Summary

Drive when you are honestly capable. You are not your own best judge. Seek advice on the level of safety and competency with which to operate a car, bicycle, motorcycle, skateboard, in-line skates, or any toy of motion.

8

Play

Fun requires energy. When a brain injury drains energy reserves for brain healing, the body makes decisions about what will and will not be accomplished. Leisure activities are the first to drop off. In a survival situation, play is a luxury without an energy budget.

Answering the question "Am I having any fun yet?" becomes doubly rhetorical. No, you are not having any fun yet. Nor do you have the energy for it.

But play is important. This chapter reminds you that a great deal of learning and repeated familiar behaviors are reinforced with fun. Play is a valuable, vital part of recovery.

Playing Is Important

Work and play balance one another, offering variety in your life. When a brain injury enters the picture, play seems to be the first to go. We seem to focus on work as the more important of the two, when forced to make a choice.

Well, play is just as important as work. It takes the same kind of cognitive energy and time. Most importantly, let us remember how children learn. They learn through play because the new brain is involved. Fun greases the wheels, but play installs learning (and remembering of old skills, too). Play is a valuable avenue for regaining and remembering skills.

Play takes a lot of energy; spare energy you may not have. Because your brain is in survival mode, it may rule out fun in favor of a nap.

Your Hobbies

Almost everyone has a hobby, activity, sport, pastime, or intriguing avocation that captures their attention and imagination. Though you may not have time to fully satisfy your inclination in this direction, I strongly recommend that you take even 10 minutes weekly to practice the enjoyment you receive from this hobby.

You may discover, to your disappointment, that your hobby no longer holds interest for you. This is temporary. You are just too tired, melancholic, and overwhelmed to make room for it in your brain. Give yourself time. The charm of it will return.

Fun

What do you do for fun now? Has fun been put on the back burner in favor of staring off into space? Well, this too shall pass.

Is it tiring thinking of fun things to do? In that case, let someone else plan some fun for you. You be in charge of the boundaries: time, location, duration, topic. Even a few laughs will lift your spirits. Laughing triggers endorphins, the brain's "happy" chemicals. Endorphins are very beneficial for healing.

Something as easy as having someone make popcorn and rent a video for you can be considered fun at this stage of the game. Fun is important. Laughter is important. Figuring out what is fun for you now is paramount.

Am I having fun yet? You may discover that having fun is an effort, and that it can actually make you angry, agitated, resentful, and overwhelmed. Fun may happen too fast, be too loud, be jarring, be annoying. This is all OK. It will pass.

That's Not Funny

Laughter takes energy, just like work. The key is to find a balance that provides you with a few laughs while not tiring you out.

You Need a Vacation

Is going on vacation the last thing you see yourself doing? Is the thought of planning, packing, organizing, and even departing too much to handle? That sounds about right. A vacation may be a useful recovery goal. Work up to it.

It took me a year to be able to go on a vacation that was actually a vacation. A basic, one-stop, one-step vacation such as an all-inclusive format works very well with brain injury, particularly if you alert the management ahead of time to your special needs. Specific planning and a no-fuss destination add to the success.

AUGUST 6, 1992 BREAKFAST IN THE RAIN

We awoke to that famous Northwest drizzle. Hard to distinguish from the Nooksack River, rushing by in its milkiness, headed for the Falls.

It smells like rain, and spots of wet ground are visible from the folds of the tent. The picnic table is accumulating mini-puddles of precipitation. Good morning in the North Cascades. As we lie in our cozy bags torn between snuggling and the call of Mother Nature, we survey the new options of the day, which now do not include Plan A: hiking around Mt. Shuksan and Mt. Baker. We list our options to the melody of droplets and fir needles as the tent catches them on their way to earth.

To dress, scurry, and emerge from the tent, having performed all rolling and stuffing duties prior, is a fine-tuned skill of the wet camp. Then, off to nature's call, returning to fold the tent.

Dining in the car seems the driest forum available. Out comes shredded wheat. Sprinkle wild blueberries. Pour on the 2%, which tastes like cream to the fat and cholesterol counters, and driving the spoon into the giant camping bowl, the freshly harvested capsules of blue sweet delight bob and swim, outnumbering the wheat shreds, showering more frosting than cake in this amazing gift from the hillsides of yesterday's hike.

As crowning touch, we find a classical station on the radio, so amid Beethoven, Saint Saens, and history of the Boston Philharmonic, we gleefully consume our bowls of Mountain Treasure, fogging up the windows and slurping that final gulp of twilight-shaded milk from the bowl.

This bowl, however, being a bit bigger than the bowls at home, where the art of slurping is practiced in office garb at the dining table, this toss of the cream overmatches its mark and decorates not only the lips, but chin and aqua Patagonia to boot.

No finer testimony to a chef than the grin of satisfaction upon the blue and white lips of the happy camper whilst completing a perfect meal.

Exercise

What does it take to get you moving? Are you used to exercise? Did you consider yourself an active person? Does exercise "move too fast" for you now? Has exercise disappeared from your daily routine? Are you just too tired and overwhelmed to get moving? Is the gym a noisy, overwhelming, intimidating place?

Think about what you used to do for exercise. Did you walk, ride bikes, ski, do yoga, do aerobics, lift weights, jog, dance, hike, in-line skate, play softball, bowl, or swim? What percentage of your former activity are you honestly participating in now?

FEBRUARY 17, 1993: GETTING EXERCISE

Before the accident, nothing could keep me off the slopes, off the trails, out of the gym, or away from fun. I was a lean, trim, stretched, and strong outdoorsy kinda gal.

With the accident came a lot of rest, required eating, and recovery. A little walking, around the block at first, was my exercise. And 25 pounds of protection added to my frame. Getting back to the groove has been a major challenge. And I don't feel totally back yet.

Sustaining regular exercise has been difficult. In the early recovery days, walking partners were regular and steady. Once I returned to work and my limited wardrobe of what still fit, regular exercise gave way to mental fatigue and depression.

False start after false start, coupled with all the "shoulds" and the tight-waisted reminders were no help. Even a Nordic Track parked in the living room was not motivating enough.

Finally, the Pilates Method and my friend Jane, who teaches it, came along. Whether it's the gentle success of the Pilates or the support of the instructor, I've actually gone regularly. It feels like success to just show up somewhere on a consistent basis. My body is growing stronger. My waistline is still the same, but my self-esteem has risen tremendously.

Get an Exercise Buddy

One hurdle that became clear to me as I tried to get back on the exercise horse was that I was intimidated and afraid of failure. The issue of "initiation" was never more clear to me than with exercise. I could not seem to get out the door to the gym on my own. I needed a reason outside myself to get it done.

Without the outside commitment to another person or class, no sheer force of will was working. My singular efforts were all short term, and filled with disappointing outcomes and disappointing results. I became a failure in my own eyes, especially because my life had been so exercise centered. Now, it seemed, I could not even go by myself for a walk around the block in broad daylight.

My failure to exercise chewed away at my fragile self-esteem. I could not even exercise with the television hard bodies in the privacy of my own home. I felt doomed. I felt agoraphobic. I thought I was becoming afraid to leave the house. Another thing to worry about.

The key was to connect my exercise to another person or class so that I was expected to show up. Once another person entered the picture, whether or not he knew that he was my exercise buddy, I became more able to keep the commitment. This not only got me out of the initiation loop (because I was no longer the source of the activity in my own mind), it got me out of the house.

Once I got out of the house and on the way to the activity, I was back in the exercise saddle again. (Having dogs that you have to walk, even if they are someone else's dogs, can commit you to a daily routine.)

It Wasn't Always Pretty

There were times when I was exercising that I would burst into tears, become emotional, feel nauseous, want to run away, want to quit, or want to just go home. Sometimes I toughed it out, and sometimes I did go home. The key was to be gentle with myself. I offered no judgment and remembered that this would take perseverance.

There were times when I felt no real goal accomplishment with exercise. Sometimes I felt fat and unattractive (usually just before my period, which was off schedule). When I would remind myself of the healing process chart and the aspects of progress, plateau, and refuel, it smoothed the feelings.

Exercise can be too noisy, too fast, too active, too complicated, too sequential, too scary, and too emotional an experience. Some days are fun. Some days you just put in your time and wait for the cumulative effect to kick in. On occasion, just go home early.

Just keep showing up. Parts of you will catch up eventually. And in the meantime, the fresh air is beneficial.

Be a Kid

Remember how much fun it was to play as a kid? Remember that teacher who figured out a way to offer you fun and learning at the same time? Well, the more "child" you can bring to your fun, the more you will be able to remember. Repeating old skills, things you did as a kid, is a great pattern refresher for your brain. You not only may repeat and reinforce what you know (that might be locked up inside), you may actually have fun in the process.

Swimming is a great refresher. Start with a plastic wading pool in your yard. Just have fun, cool your feet, watch how many little kids spontaneously show up. Hand out a few squirt guns and wind-up shark toys and have a great time. Then graduate to the swimming pool and splash around. Swim a few laps, do a little back float, hold your breath, and blow bubbles underwater. (If this activity proves too overstimulating, back off to a calmer yet still gleeful level, and build from there.)

It might seem pedestrian at first, but the truth is you do remember how to swim. It is very good for your self-esteem and you'll have fun.

Exercise Restores Self-Esteem

Accomplishment has a way of restoring self-esteem. When you begin to experience "Yes, I can" once again, it makes a tremendous difference. The freedom to be in the world again seems to have returned. The mind releases itself from pain and partakes in the positive beauty of life. This is good.

Of course, I headed for Utah. The exercise of walking, hiking, camping, and traveling was having a positive effect upon my demeanor and outlook. I was getting my life back.

APRIL 1992

Ten days on the road with the ones we love. Doing the desert thing. Tourists in the dust. Seeking the high cracks, the blossoms of the desert in spring, the ultimate stillness of the lonesome rock, the deep quiet of the caves and shade.

The shade, 30 degrees cooler than the direct, ozone-thin sunshine. The shade, where the bats leave evidence of their overnight camping. The sunlight, where the first, south-facing, protected spots harbor a prickly armload of Claret Cups, those wine-red cactus that lead the spring parade.

Springtime heat and springtime snow, springtime dust, and sprinkle. The first of the lace-winged midges ("no-see-em's" to you) makes her moisture-seeking appearance at dusk, locating your nose, eyes, mouth, and ears faster than your two hands can wave her off. It seems unfair that this announcement of dinnertime should arrive before the full bloom of the desert floor. Too much rain last summer. Too hardy. They outsmarted us this year. With their early appearance, and the welts they leave behind in the hairline and other very soft spots. Lumps that may last a week, left by a creature too small to swat.

We sit at the foot of the Super Crack, a small stop on the way to our third campsite. We have already chased our tent in wind and snow in the shadow of Castleton Tower. Strolled at the feet of the Fisher King and Titan Tower and the Ancient Art Wall. Walked a path well worn by the faithful and the curious to Delicate Arch, filled our jugs with water at the legendary Matrimony Springs, and braved the crowds at City Market in Moab on Easter Sunday.

Now we leave the Needles after two days of walking, climbing, and soaking in the great stillness that desert wilderness offers.

Far different than the mountains, rivers, oceans, and forests of the earth, desert silence speaks to a still part within me that makes room for more peace and serenity. There is a silence here not found elsewhere. A silence so profound one must come to terms with oneself or either go mad or crank the tunes to keep the noise level sufficient so as to most efficiently block the inner messages; the evidence of resolution unbaked.

Summary

Moving your body is vital to the restoration of cranial function. Fresh air, activity, laughter, elevated heart rate, and a change of scenery are good for the body, mind, and spirit. You know this part. Just do it.

9

Sexual Response

When the brain is injured, it prioritizes its energy for survival. Energy from "less-vital" parts of the brain is somehow sent to help out in the injured area. Pleasure centers are less vital than visual, breathing, or decision centers, for example. So, you may feel lethargic or uninterested in going to the movies or a party. Sexual response is not vital to short-term survival. It is another area that becomes turned down or off until the energy levels return and it can be "funded" again. Very often the hypothalamus, which regulates desire and sex hormones, is involved in the brain injury. This results in changes in your sexual response.

Sexual arousal, pleasure from stimulation, or even orgasm may be difficult or nonfunctional for a while. Hugging and hand holding might be the extent of it. Kissing may be affected as well. You may become tactilely defensive and unable to tolerate being touched. Fortunately, there are other ways of being close.

This chapter discusses sexual response. And, yes, it is like a bicycle. You will remember how to do it. I hope you find this information useful and reassuring.

Sex

Because of the brain injury, the sexual parts of your body may not respond the way you may be used to them responding. You may be overwhelmed by sexual response just now. Also, you may be unable to deal with "large doses" of intimate contact. Moderating and beginning slowly are key. Arousal may be slow or unapparent at first. Frustration over lack of response may eat away at your self-esteem. Fear not. Your brain just is not ready for this activity yet. Also, you may see yourself differently and may not feel like a sexually desirable person yet. Be gentle with yourself, and take all the time you need.

External Modeling

When I practice a behavior that is not automatic, but that I used to be able to perform, I call this process "external modeling." As I experience this way of reminding the brain of what it already knows, I simply go through the motions of the unremembered behavior. What I notice while practicing this method of remembering is that my brain picks up bits and pieces of the behavior and re-remembers the behavior.

External modeling is not a perfect concept, but, in fits and starts, the memory can be reminded and reactivated back to the remembered behavior. I tried this idea on sexual response.

Even though the thrill was gone from kissing, and my breasts seemed unresponsive, my partner and I kissed anyway and caressed anyway. We held one another and fondled and snuggled and made love. Sometimes there was a response, but at first there was rarely a recognizable or orderly response.

Almost Orgasm

I cannot count the number of times an orgasm eluded me. Sex is, simply put, a tension-release experience. It involves a great deal of energy as well as momentum. Being short on energy and momentum, I would just run out of gas before I could get to the top of the hill, so to speak.

During the next stage of recovery, when orgasm became an occasional occurrence, many times I thought I was going to have a heart attack. Chest pain and excessively rapid breathing took over. It scared me.

Your Aerobic Rate

Sex in small doses is very important. Your cardiovascular system may have experienced a sympathetic disturbance of your aerobic ability. Your aerobic rate may be reduced by temporary changes in your body, triggered by biochemical body reactions. In other words, when your head is injured, your overall energy is reduced. This may be reflected in your heart rate. Your active, aerobic ability may be reduced.

So, if your heart is beating too fast for the conditions, back off. You are not ready. It could take your heart an average of one year to begin to increase its aerobic capacity again. Remember, this is not about your ability to have sex or about your previous level of physical fitness. This is about a part of brain injury. With time, this piece should improve.

Do not try to hop the barrier. Like your brain, your heart is in cahoots with your energy system and will slow you down. Listen to your heart. This is not about achievement or advanced physical performance. It is about listening to your body. You need a balanced, intelligent adherence to moderate guidelines, which maintain a healthy body. It is vital that you guard against taxing or depleting your energy supply.

Of course, you want to be able to have sex again. Slow, measured, and moderate steps are called for here. Practice is good. To be overwhelmed during practice can sap your energy. The time it takes each person to restore his energy differs. And the emotional trials during the wait can take their toll. Then, one day, it seems to be better. Here's what the journal says:

JANUARY 8, 1993

> Finally, the sex is better! Or rather, back to good, on its way back to great. Inflated memory notwithstanding, my sexual response has been missing a few chips lately.
>
> Is it the lower blood supply from not having a spleen? The brain injury (sex being 90% in your head)? The distant drum of menopause steadily and relentlessly tromping my way? The depression? My partner? (No way, he is a hunk.) Too long out of the saddle?
>
> And since one of my vivid memories that served me all too well was the energetic life I had led occasionally, at least in my mind, I wondered.
>
> So what could be wrong? First answer: there is something wrong with me.
>
> Well, maybe so. Maybe I lost that, too. But something told me to just stick with it. Go through the motions, enjoy the loving contact, and maybe repetition would restore the pathways

or make new ones. And the practice wasn't too bad in the meantime.

So I stuck with it, watching, noticing, occasionally experiencing a "real" orgasm (you know the difference), many times just skipping over the top of a climax without an actual release. As if it could get just so far, then disappear into the mist.

My erogenous zones did not seem connected either. Used to be any breast or nipple manipulation sent me on a trip to the light fantastic. That was gone. And my vaginal moisture was inconsistent in response. That's when we discovered Astro Glide. My ears were no longer erotically connected and my mouth had returned only to a "meaningful smooth" level of intensity. The wires seemed disconnected, yet visible. What to do? Just keep loving.

With a loving and caring partner, last night my nipples worked again! They actually tingled! Yahoo! Another part fixed. That tingle made its way all the way to those magical spots, somewhere under the soft curly pillow. If we can get that far, let's make my toes tingle, too. Well, back to practice.

The subtle pieces of one's rocked life strangely seem the most important. Regaining the most private pieces amount to the greatest, though largely unnoticed, victories. Another glimmer of hope on the trail of cranial recovery.

Kind of makes becoming lost and overshooting my destination by 10 miles to a place I have been numerous times seem normal. Everybody gets turned around. I got my nipples back today. Another layer lifted (my neurologist is going to crack up when she reads this book).

Tingling

When feelings of sexual response began to return for me, I identified the feeling as "tingling." It was almost two years before this pleasure returned. Here is the journal entry:

FEBRUARY 1, 1993

I finally tingled. A year of intimate practice and lots of warm-fuzzy but unsatisfying evenings, and I finally tingled! Not only that, but a little flush and sweat (do ladies sweat?) to my skin as well. Yes! Another piece of recovery evidence.

Self-diagnosis was inconclusive. (We all know what Abraham Lincoln said about representing yourself in court!) Abdominal trauma? No, I still had regular periods. No spleen, no sheen? No, working out and climbing 14,000-ft. peaks made sweat. Complicated brain task with lots of sequencing? Most likely a combination of everything? Maybe. Nothing left to do but keep practicing to see what changed or got better. Lubrication is improving, too, as is nipple sensitivity. Sure would be great to get the triple orgasms back. Every recovery has its ultimate carrot.

Sex Could Be Different

Just as you may need to find new pathways to information stored in your brain, so too may you need to discover new pleasure pathways. Sex may just be different now. Orgasm may feel different to you, may happen in different ways, through a different rhythm, or may even be located in different "places." Also, be aware that some medications can alter your sexual response, particularly certain antidepressants. Consult your doctor about side effects of your medication.

Exploration within a supportive relationship is most helpful. Remember, however, that there is value in self-exploration. If you are without an intimate partner at this time, self-pleasure and self-appreciation are most reasonable. The idea of external modeling still applies here.

Remember, it's hard to feel sexual when you are exhausted. Any new parent can verify that experience. Plan for sexual activity when you are the most rested. Your experience may be less spontaneous than desired, but it does hedge the odds that you will have enough energy to enjoy yourself.

Universal Precautions Note

Vulnerability can be an issue for the affection-starved, brain-injured person. Remember, safe sex. No glove, no love. The last thing you need is a sexually transmitted disease to further tax your limited energy supply and weakened immune system.

Couples Issues: You and Your Partner

Relationship and intimacy issues can stress any partnership. Brain injury complicates relationship. With a strong, committed relationship, patience and practice will conquer a lot. If your relationship was on thin ice to begin with, you (and most specifically your uninjured partner) may need support to survive your recovery. (See the chapter "For Family Members.")

You will likely experience moments, days, weeks, or more of irritability. This is normal because your brain injury is annoying to your nervous system and can make you grumpy. It will pass, but it is not an enhancing feature of relationships! Acknowledge up front that there will be "moments," and work with your partner to establish common goals of kindness, compassion, patience, appreciation, and forgiveness.

Education for your partner on brain-injury issues will help as well. Enroll one another in the process and the journey. Commit to the sustainability of your relationship and the positive outcomes reached together with gentle understanding and mutual vision.

Girl Talk

Although this section is written for women, it will be helpful for men to read it also. The circadian rhythm of the body, for both men and women, can be seriously impacted with brain injury. You can easily feel out of sorts, or out of step. Biochemically, your entire being has been affected. Men, as well as women, may find themselves in this section.

JANUARY 28, 1993

> Let's talk hormones, cycles, insomnia, and the munchies. It makes me nervous when my period does not start on time. Not for the usual reason. The PMS clock just winds tighter and tighter while it waits. Maybe edgy is a better word; bitchy. That captures the true essence.
>
> But, hey, when the forces of nature are disrupted, it takes a while to calm the waters, so to speak. For those of us on the "moon cycle" (that's 13 periods per year), we flow every 29 days or so. And the pull of the full moon or the ease of the new moon attracts most of us.
>
> Trauma can delay or interrupt a cycle. In my case, a week in the hospital moved me to start a week after the full moon. For the next 1–1/2 years, the cycle attempted to readjust itself by working its way through the phases of the moon until it came full circle, then overshot the new moon again.
>
> Today it's a few days past the old starting date and may go through the correction cycle again. Definitely makes for uncertain PMS times.

Staying alert to physiologic changes helped me track it, but having tender breasts for two weeks gets old fast.

For those of us who also are wide awake one night a month, this lasted two days sometimes. Comes with the territory. Even with the caffeine/alcohol/processed meat/sugar/Nutrasweet/MSG/Splenda-free diet. Even with the B6, lecithin, vitamin complex, bulk- and fiber-laden, chocolate-free, exercise, and lots of water advantages. Add in the acupressure, hot tub, and conscious munching.

It's the best I could do. My cycle was seeking a balance.

For a while I thought it was menopause. Spotting, extra bitchiness, "feminine itching," poor sexual lubrication, swollen body parts, depression, lethargy, hair loss, shortness of humor. I even bought menopause books, checked my family history, and went to the gynecologist.

My brain was just shopping for balance. That took three to four months before it subsided. The cycle has settled down some now, but it is still creeping forward on the calendar.

The things I used to crave have changed, too. Used to be graham crackers, bread, wheat foods, chocolate. Now there are oat bran crackers, popcorn, corn chips, potatoes, black beans. No transition period.

As with all things, listen to your body. She is telling you something that you may not understand, but, try as you might, nothing else satisfies like the request. Nurture yourself.

Hypersexuality

If your brain injury includes frontal disinhibition (an injury aspect that relieves you of your ability to discern appropriate social behaviors), you may experience hypersexuality and turn into a rabbit. The potential for "raping" your partner is present. Should you have rabbit feelings about your partner, bring it to the attention of your psychotherapist and your partner immediately.

Summary

Lack of sexual response is a temporary casualty of the recovery process and usually returns within one year. It is not vital to your immediate survival, though it may be vital to your personal identity. Be very gentle with your body, your participation in moderate activity, and with your partner. You can quickly deplete your energy pie with sexual activity. Slowly, gently, and lovingly proceed.

10

Re-entry

When enough parts of the You that you remember come back, there may be this feeling of relief and "Yes, I'm back." That may be a good time for a journey back to learning. Testing out your learning skills is extremely important. As human beings, we never really stop learning.

Your learning style may have changed within your recovery. You need to know as much about your learning style as possible so that you can continue to succeed in your daily life.

This chapter is about learning to learn again. We will focus upon remembering what you know about learning, as well as possible differences between your present learning style and your previous experience with learning.

JANUARY 18, 1992

> I'm emerging out the other side of the haze, the curtain, that fog of cranial recovery so dim and relentless you think you've been driving for days in a ground blizzard. Neck forward as if getting that much closer to the windshield would really make a difference. Hands so firmly on the steering wheel, the ache of the grasp digs deeply into shoulders and hips. Eyes so intently on the unavailable scenery, they dart about, fixing on nothing, desperately seeking anything.
>
> Emerging. Slowly. I recognize myself for the most part. I can go to work now. But I'm restless. I can ski, but I forget a few parts. Not all the people who know me are familiar. The faces ring a

bell. The names are in some database in a locked room in my head. Usually the key is provided by the face.

It isn't as embarrassing anymore to simply say "I bumped my head, and the card with your name on it got flipped into the snow. Please tell me your name.

So, the fog is lifting. The world is becoming more accessible, more palpable. This is good. This is a great time to explore. This is also a great time for a relapse because re-entry will be a surprise to your system. Just thought I would mention that.

Learning to Learn Again

Human beings take information into their brains generally one of three ways: they see it (visual), they hear it (auditory), or they touch it (kinesthetic). There is debate whether smell (sensory) is a fourth way. Intuitive or emotional learning (feeling) is a fifth way. At the least, the last two are influential.

This is how we learn. Show me, tell me, let me touch it, let me feel it, let me take it in. We all tend to be dominant in one of these areas and receive secondary information from the others. Do you know which way you learn? Now is a good time to find out.

Do you say: I hear what you are saying? I see what you are saying? I can put my finger on what you are saying? I can smell that one a mile away? It is a simple test, but it will help you tremendously to discover how you learn best.

Once you know your dominant information conduit, you can frame learning so that you will perceive and understand.

I am mostly visual. Give me a map. Telling me directions goes in one ear and out the other. *See* what I mean? As you learn to learn again, give yourself the best possible advantage. Try to orient new information to your recognized primary sensory model. Frame new information so you can take it in most effectively.

Take a Class

Someday you will want to understand and test your capacities. It may be time for you to enroll in a class that interests you and where no one will know you. You can discover and experience your abilities in privacy while doing something fun. Talk to your instructor at the very beginning about any special accommodation. Something as simple as a quiet room to take a test, or moving you away from the furnace ducts so you can hear better, can make all the difference to your success.

A class will help you sort out how you learn. It will also remind you that you can learn. Success and fun are satisfying reinforcers. General knowledge, conduct in a group, and asking for and receiving support are all excellent for the ego. Being there as a stranger will remind you that the world is an accessible place and you are SUCCEEDING in it!

When I signed up for weaving, I wanted to practice sequencing, cross-crawling, fun, and learning in an anonymous group. It worked.

Re-Entry Can Be Scary

MAY 6, 1993: THE TRUTH IS NO EXCUSE

So when is it that the brain injury stops being your story, excuse, explanation, place to hide? It's embarrassing, but when I feel cornered or pressured or stuck or challenged, I have begged off or sought sympathy. It's tacky, it's esteem eroding and it's true.

So I had a brain injury. How long will I keep using the "truth" as my excuse? Yes, it's a bummer, yes I get tired, yes it's a big challenge to grow. But at what point does my excuse become an ethical challenge? How broad are the skirts behind which we hide? And for how long?

Letting go is hard work. Hard work is good. Do it. If you get tired, just do it in smaller chunks.

APRIL 12, 1993: I CAN WORK AGAIN

Today the breakthrough was quiet and relieving. A regular work day, but no clients. So I began proofreading the first draft of this book. At home. Worked in the living room. Spread out the notes with their yellow swipes of highlighter pointing out the unintelligible words for me to fill in on the draft. Spread out the draft on my lap.

Read, corrected, filled in, fixed sentences, added more stuff. Made tea, did a load of laundry. Answered the phone. Made a few calls. And did not turn on the TV. In fact, didn't have an interest in watching. And there it was, across the living room. Standing silent vigil to my cognitive resting needs.

Today, what I was doing pulled me strongly, held my attention, fascinated me, intrigued me, and kept me focused. Today I kicked the TV habit. The next phase of my recovery has arrived.

I am in charge now. Not the TV. It does not call me away from my work. My brain is no longer seeking conscious naps. My attention span has finally reached a critical level of sustainability.

Yes! The concentration barrier has been broken. Focus and continuous attention is possible again. It is a strong feeling. An endurance feeling. A reclaiming of power. I can work again!

When I Attended the Writer's Workshop

As part of a workshop I attended in Utah, we were each granted audience with our instructor. Susan Tweit, a published naturalist, was my instructor. We were to submit a writing sample and have it reviewed. This is my journal entry of that meeting.

NOVEMBER 8, 1992

She liked my work. No, she said it brought tears to her eyes. My journal entry. She said I spoke straight. That my issues touched her. That publishing was a good idea. That my style is workable. That proceeding is a good idea. That she encourages me to stop by her home in New Mexico.

She is interested in my work and wants me to keep in touch on my progress. That makes me feel very good. Respected. Encouraged. Validated. I feel like cream rising to the top. There are no illusions here. A lot of work ahead. More bridges to cross. More remembering who I am.

The journal continues:

Today I remembered myself again. The confidence I came searching for is not what I found. In its place is a warmer, expanded piece of silent space inside—a comfortable, familiar, almost intimate feeling of inner recall. As if the door were opened and I walked in warmly greeted, my coat taken, led to the banquet hall as an expected and warmly anticipated guest. I seem to be wearing a long black and red gown, simple diamond choker, and sensible flats concealed by the sculpted hemline as it brushes the marble hallway.

Gliding to a high-backed chair, graciously held for my descending, slinky buns, a sumptuous vichyssoise with triangle bread crusts smothered in an asparagus butter are set before me. I reach for the Chardonnay and gaze above the rim of the goblet seeking unobtrusive eye contact over the oaky bouquet.

Then reality returns. Slurred words came back today. Mud slide, mud slide. My man would whisper his sensory overload theory gently in my direction, and I would remember that the healing is still not finished.

Better, but not done. Another piece of the depression has lifted. Creativity has come back. Thoughts flow more freely. I remember how term papers used to roll off my fingertips, first draft. How concepts, outlines, introductions, and conclusions lined up in my head awaiting manual discharge through the typewriter keys.

I notice how that insistent delivery style has returned. How sentences write themselves on the inside of my head, reverberating in the cranial cavern until the ears hear it from the inside, until the elves in my eyes write the words like a layer in the optic jelly, forcing me to see the thoughts, read the words: The only release from this torture is placing pen to paper and unlocking those phrases held captive and creating such a racket.

Yes, this looks like recovery to me. Feeling compelled, driven, and passionate about anything feels more like the old me. But, of course, you didn't know the "old me." Truthfully, I had less than a full grip on her either. Always busy, always producing, striving, creating, going, coming, hiking, skiing, working, reading, playing, scheming for vacations. Driven. Driven by illusion masters. Focused but goalless. Talented, with limited maps of the area. Task oriented but empty.

A bright, energetic, loving, and loved individual with all the external signs of having my scat in a pile.

Looking for love in all the right places. Successful under the circumstances. Confident, funny, brash, professional, trusted, and loved. A great cook, creative wit, and exceptional problem solver. Able to keep houseplants green and happy. Able to keep dear friends for the long haul. Detail oriented with a certain knack for long-term vision and projection. Slim and trim. Energetic. Health conscious. Lots of mountain trips. Fresh air a must.

I lived in a whirlwind. And when that whirlwind came to an abrupt halt, part of me was missing when I woke up.

Parts of me are still missing, but as I hunt for those last little bits (like looking for the back of an earring popped off your ear by taking off a sweater, then down on hands and knees hoping for that telltale metallic flash that whispers "over here" among the carpet fibers, trying to ignore the surface dust that hovers in your nostrils as you eyeball the floor and ignore the dust bunnies in the defocused range of sight), I remember the pieces found to date and finally know that stragglers will continue to trickle in. That I am finally OK just as I am today.

Oh, how many times have I given that phrase as homework to my clients, only to need to hear it with my own ears, my own heart, my own being now. Have I finally come to practice what I preach—to listen, as well, to these great and simple words.

To simply love myself each day. To remember what I can remember on any given day and to let it be enough.

To allow my exhausted and overworked brain a rest. To simply go to bed and snuggle and let that simple act of love and contact remind me that I am still loved, even on this side of the story, that this one quality sustains and nourishes me. That through it all, I have remained loving and lovable. The sense of peace is complete for today. I have remembered that I am loved. Suddenly it seems easier to breathe.

What I have to say is of value to others. My presence is of value. I can contribute in confidence again. The feeling is back.

Declare New Life

All in all, declaring that you have a new life is a good idea. Wallowing in what used to be takes valuable time and energy you cannot spare. Discover for yourself that you are new, fresh, and lovable. Get going.

DECEMBER 23, 1992

Sometimes I feel like I've fallen over and I can't reach myself. Who I used to be.

It's time to say good-bye. To who I was. To who I may never be again. It's entirely possible that I won't ever be the old me again. There are plenty of good things about the new me. Maybe it's time to give her a chance. A chance to grow up and experience life. Maybe I'm not 43. Perhaps I'm a mere 1–1/2.

Keep Trying

Some days are harder to live through than others. Some days work well. Other days stretch my energy limits. Some days are meant for just showing up.

Just put in the time. It won't necessarily show on the credit side of the ledger today, but it will contribute to the overall result. After all, 85% of life is just showing up. Some days are just for punching the clock. So just punch the clock. You don't have to engage in deep, profound thought or progress every day.

DECEMBER 21, 1991

Saturday. Solstice. Shortest day of the year. The full moon set over the Flatirons at sunrise. Magnificent. Blazing moon. Twilight sky. Flaming red rock and the morning star framed it as it passed from sight turning an iridescent pink from the sun-risen smog cloud over Denver.

Brilliant. Crisp, clean air. Surreal moment in time. I wondered what it would have looked like in the Utah desert. Or out at sea. Or through your eyes.

So we went skiing. Loveland Mountain. The snow was challenging. Icy and shaved. Too many rocks, willows, not enough snow. A klutz day for me. Put in the mileage. Pound my thighs. Phone it in. Couldn't hold an edge. Oh well, just enjoy the view, the air, the view again. Be among friends. Do my best. The sun will be here longer from now on.

Spirit Connection

Where does the fuel come from now? A contemplative entry asks a question.

OCTOBER 24, 1992

I am different now, after all. Life's little priorities have changed. There's more private time, hardly any frantic time. The overall stress is down tremendously. Perhaps that stress fueled me for so long I measured my success by the necessary stress level.

Now, to succeed and let the stress melt away. It is not needed. Do I miss it? Did I define myself by it before? How to redefine, deepen the progress, and use another fuel. Would "spirit" fuel me? I'll check that out.

Be Present, Do Your Best, Be on Your Own Team

One day at a time and one step at a time. If the steps seem too big, just apply the being overwhelmed theory and break them into smaller steps.

Let go of the past, and be present for your new life today. It takes less energy and supports your healing process. ***You have a new life, a new start, and a new point of view.*** Aside from classic movies, where else do you get the chance at a script like that?

Be on your own team. You don't have to be the captain of the team, but you do have to show up every day for practice. Be present for yourself.

JULY 2, 1991

But back to business. Do I really want my life back? All of it? Aren't there just a few things I'd prefer differently since I'm on my second chance? Since I have it to do differently, would I?

Well, frankly, yes. There are a few items so far. Like grinding my teeth at night. Worrying . . . about anything. Withholding affection. Thinking I'm not enough, even when chained to the couch. Being as clear as possible. Asking for what I need. Pausing to think out an answer, or to relish a question. I could quit tailgating (my most heinous crime). I would like to explore another line of work. Writing, mostly. There must be more writing.

Perhaps the approach, the state of mind, of being is truly more at hand here than a shopping list of born-again dos and don'ts. It's not like I'll promise to not rob banks since I talked to God. More that I promise to talk to Spirit more, to be present for myself more. To live in the deep breath of appreciation and gratitude. Not in a gloppy, gushy way. But to just be joyful. To just be peaceful. Not like a bumper sticker quoting trite fuzzies.

To be at peace. To know that the secret of life is also the secret of death. To live and to pass on consciously. Not to walk around half-stoned on life to the exclusion of present action.

Precisely, present action. Conscious present awareness. Focused, clear, peaceful presence. Be here now, dude. Like, show up. Account for yourself. Stand and deliver.

We can do that here. That's my opportunity. Be who I fully wish to be. Give it a shot. And if you're not quite done, maybe you'll be sent back to polish it up a bit; rethink, revamp, or get a secret mission.

Who knows why? But why spend time on that question when other more useful questions pop immediately into mind, such as

○　　How to modify my belly dancing costume so as not to sunburn my scar?

○　　Will I ever enjoy chicken livers again?

○   Will I climb a 14'er this season?
○   Can I stop telling my rollerblading story soon?
○   Will I really miss late-night TV once I can read again?
○   Is sex considered an aerobic use of the abdominal muscles?

These and other stirring questions are just that.

What I've mostly learned, to date, is that if you can let go of your death, everything else becomes amazingly simple and straightforward by comparison. No kidding. No kidding.

Summary

Learning, whether it is in the classroom or any room of your house, is important to your healing process. Brain training, life training, decision making, and getting on with your life are all a part of re-entry.

Do your best every day. Remember that you are OK just the way you are every minute of the day and in everything you do, say, try, or contemplate. Show up for your life, however you choose to do that. Don't wait for your life to turn out. This is your life. Be here now.

11

Travel

Travel is my favorite. Trips anywhere. Short overnights. A week on the road. Three weeks overseas to Turkey, India, Ireland. Life is planning one great adventure after another!

Your brain injury goes with you on vacation, so there are some considerations.

Travel can be overwhelming, overstimulating, and taxing. New experiences, though fabulous, take some integration time for your brain. Good fun is stressful, too. Be gentle with yourself and enjoy your mobility.

Handy Travel Tips

Good planning and strategic scheduling are key. Research your trip. Plan to travel during the daytime. Rest at night. Avoid "red eye" flights. Schedule manageable activities and touring. Compensate for changes in time zones.

Include rest days or quieter activities. (Travel, rest, travel, rest.) Avoid crowds. Travel off season if possible. Plan your biggest activities for the morning. Nap after lunch. Plan a short activity before supper. Relax.

Pack light. One suitcase, one shoulder bag. You can do it.

Carry your own water bottle. Buy your snacks along the way. (Believe me, every state or country on the planet sells snacks!) Just take a few locking plastic bags with you for easy storage and access.

Ear plugs. Great for the plane, the car, the hotel, large crowds. Take two pair. Consider taking personal music, too. People will leave you be if you are relaxing with your headphones on. And think about wearing sunglasses on the plane. Cuts down the glare, and gives you privacy!

Sensible shoes. Light jacket or sweater for taking naps on the train or bus. Hat with a brim to cut glare from the sun and overhead lights.

Eat light. Avoid alcohol, lots of caffeine, and processed foods. Remember to keep your nutrition regimen. Good fuel for your body and brain are key to maintaining your stamina.

Summary

Have a wonderful time. Notice that you are in the world, doing just fine. Before you know it, you'll be planning your next adventure!

12

Parenting and Couples Issues

Parenting

Parenting your children while healing a brain injury is a critical and difficult task. Your children need you as you were, while you are struggling to stay afloat. It is imperative to ensure that your children get the care and supervision they require. It is most important that your children not transition into the adults in your family.

This delicate dance of healing and parenting is possible with cooperation and support.

Tell Your Kids the Truth

It is imperative that you reveal to your kids (to their level of understanding) that you have a brain injury. Euphemisms or cutesy descriptions are inappropriate and disrespect your child's ability to handle the truth. Kids are smart. They know when they are being snowed. They know when you trust them enough to tell them the straight-up truth.

The truth isn't an anatomy lesson. The truth is: daddy can't drive the car just now; mommy needs your help. Answer all their questions honestly. Daddy may be a little different, and he will gain some new skills and may lose others.

The road ahead for our family will be different. We need each other now more than ever, and we will be relying on each other more. We will all be asked to do chores, errands, and household duties more than before. We hope for the best, with everyone's valuable participation.

Your Dysfunctional Household

So if you were dysfunctional, boundariless, inconsistent, partially present, and chaotic parents before your brain injury, you will have even less control now.

Whole-family guidance is in order for your family to survive. Resetting the boundaries, reestablishing authority and respect for all members of the family unit, and restoring cooperation are crucial. Your family members must be pulling in the same direction to weather this brain injury. Find a proactive and qualified family therapist who connects with all the family members, has experience with brain injury in a family, and can assist you in building strong, cooperative, and loving relationships.

Discernment

As an adult with a brain injury, your discernment skills may be hampered, and your behavior may more closely mirror that of your children. Rather than experiencing your "inner child," you could be dragged into actually acting like a child. Although this is a clear part of brain injury, it is not supportive to solid parenting.

Your behavior may lapse into an immature temperament, displaying impulsiveness and emotions in keeping with a child or adolescent. This behavior may emerge on its own or may be triggered by conflict with your children. You may be dragged to their level instantly, mirroring their undeveloped behavior.

When this happens, and to the best of your ability, take a time-out in an adult manner to retain your kids' respect and to regain your adult composure. Reconnect with your adult center. Calm down. Agree to take up the issue at another time, preferably with your spouse or the therapist present.

Establish, with your therapist's assistance, a cue that gives you an escape from a volatile situation. This cue must be agreeable to all family members. It allows for you to temporarily remove yourself from an untenable situation, yet guarantees respect for the issue and resolution in the future for all members of the conflict.

Brain Injury and Relationships with Your Children

With some brain injuries, there is an alteration of emotional connection with people around you. Your loving connection with your children may shift temporarily. You may become disconnected or unable to empathize at first. The deep loving feeling may shift and need to find a new avenue of expression and connection.

This problem is likely temporary and a symptom of your brain injury. As your injury heals and more-complex brain function returns, your connection will likely restore itself. Report this issue to your psychotherapist for support and resolution.

Kids and School

Keeping an eye on your kids at school is important. The stress of a rearranged family dynamic may press upon their school work and social life. Track homework to ensure it is completed. Get help for your kids through a tutor or school peer helper. If you cannot contact the school personally, have a friend or your family therapist support you with this request.

For older kids and teens, especially when activities and sports are involved, work out a schedule. Kids can be very resourceful getting rides to and from events. It is OK to ask other parents for support.

Keep after-school and weekend activities at a sane level. Two activities per season is plenty. Homework comes first.

For driving teens, car rules are imperative. Driving is still a privilege and the number of kids in a car is crucial to safety. Establish a "choices and consequences" agreement with the family therapist to regulate behavior and cooperative action.

Kids and Play

If your house is the kids' congregation location, it may be important to adjust the frequency of visits and numbers of kids involved in the beginning. Have a meeting with all the kids and explain the situation. Involve the kids in the schedule-planning, snack-making, and clean-up responsibilities. Explain the necessity for lower noise levels. Go for cooperation, boundaries, and the support of their and your needs. Maybe include a homework time and another parent to drop in to help out. Kids are very inventive and will create new ways to get what they want, which is to be at your house!

Fun with Kids

Staying active and engaged with kids is important. Select activities that are fun for the kids and hold low visual and auditory impact for you. Going for ice cream, visiting a park or the zoo at off-peak hours. Walk the dog. Choose new games that kids enjoy and you can play along. Read with the kids. Make puppets. You can have plenty of fun that meets everyone's needs.

Family Meetings

Plan to meet often as a family. Discuss positive issues, make space for conflict resolution, explore new ways to amend plans, offer new strategies, and create more fun and positive support for all family members. Check in with each member to affirm that life is going along as well as possible under the circumstances. Make family meetings fun and a safe place to be.

Do not mix dinner and punishment. Mealtime is a sacred and powerful bonding event, and every member is important. Ask each member to report on a positive event from the day. (Boundaries include no phones, TV, or electronic devices at the table.)

Family Menus

The low-glycemic menu is very good for a brain-injured person. These foods are also great for kids of all ages. Essentially, it is a whole food, fresh food, moderate protein concept. Unprocessed carbohydrates and lots of delicious choices. Remember, you are the adult and you buy the food. Kids will eat what's available. When good stuff is in the house, they'll figure it out. Keep your boundaries. Be impervious to guilt trips.

Couples Issues

A supportive spouse is a blessing. Act as a team, a united front in your parenting. Work together creating a strong family. Gain suggestions from your family therapist on actions and concepts to try.

Your spouse will be taxed from extra stress. Work on your marriage communication and keep it open, honest, and loving. Come together to create and hold your relationship sacred and paramount to the success of your family story. Brain injury leans heavily upon a couple's relationship. Make time to be together. Plan a get-away overnight or weekend if possible. Restorative activities are vital to long-term strength and bonding. Be willing to fall in love again.

Consciously create a calm home atmosphere and a peaceful bedroom. Soft lighting, calm paint colors, and a decluttered environment add peace and quiet to a room. This retreat space provides a safe place when you are feeling overwhelmed, overstimulated, or in need of quiet space.

Engage the services of an organizing specialist or interior designer skilled in the ways of the peaceful home.

Be aware that there may be family-dynamic role reversals that occur between you and your spouse. Acknowledge these shifts and allow the changes. Get support if the shifts are beyond the knowledge base of the spouse. Math homework, discipline, cooking, and organizing the laundry are a few that come to mind. Give it a try. See how it goes. Get the help of your family therapist to discover more choices.

Summary

Parent as consciously as possible. Stay connected, keep your boundaries, and develop a strong team approach. Seek family therapy for fresh ideas.

"...if I only had a brain..."
Scarecrow, "Wizard of Oz"

EXECUTIVE FUNCTIONS

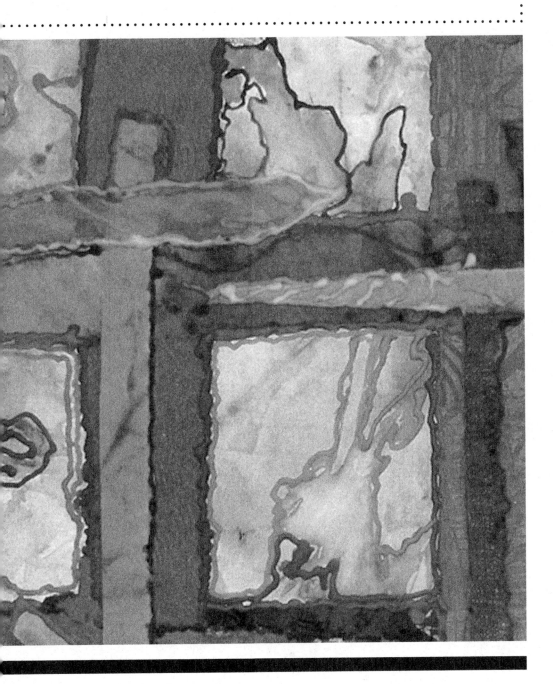

13

Executive Functions

The functions your brain performs that produce awareness, follow-through, self-motivation, self-correction, and self-initiation are considered executive functions. Lifestyle activities such as opening your mail regularly, paying bills, leading an orderly life, washing your glasses, shopping, cooking, putting on make-up, remembering, sequencing, taking a shower, and remembering to rinse the shampoo out of your hair also are included in the definition.

Multi-track thinking and the speed at which thoughts are processed are considered executive functions. This chapter discusses, individually, the various facets of "Executive Functions."

The following serves as a general overview of a tremendous amount of information. Most everything introduced here has a whole chapter written about it later. Read slowly, and feel free to focus on and branch out with one idea at a time. Executive functions are key in the brain-injury recovery process. Being overwhelmed is a normal part of reduced executive function ability. Keep breathing. Consider this description:

Unlike more severe traumatic brain injuries, the disturbance of brain function in mild traumatic brain injury (MTBI) is related more so to dysfunction of brain metabolism rather than a frank structural injury or damage. The current understanding of the underlying pathology of MTBI involves a paradigm shift away from a hardware/anatomic damage model to a software/neuronal dysfunction model, involving a complex cascade of ionic, metabolic and physiologic events. The cascade includes shifts in ionic concentrations, indiscriminate release of excitatory amino acids (glutamate), altered brain glucose metabolism (first hyperglycolysis, then hypoglycolysis), reduced cerebral blood flow, with possible axonal injury—resulting in impaired connectivity and changes in neurotransmission. Clinical signs and symptoms of MTBI such as poor attention, memory, speed of processing, and motor function are manifestations of this underlying neurometabolic cascade."[9]

Processing Speed

Does the world move too fast to you? Are you unable to hold on to more than one thought at a time? Do people speak too quickly for you? Are you unable to follow a plot or get a joke? Do you forget why you went downstairs? Do you complete your sentences? Can you anticipate the consequences of your actions? Can you decode nonverbal social cues like body language, facial expressions, and tone of voice?

You may discover that your thinking speed has slowed down. The world around you may be moving faster than you can comprehend or absorb. Life may feel like it is in slow motion, that it takes you a long time to integrate a task you previously performed quickly and efficiently.

Simple directions may not seem so simple anymore. When these are your experiences, your brain has slowed the speed with which it deals with incoming information. Your speed of processing has adjusted.

Attention Span

The period of time in which you maintain undivided attention to a task is your attention span. When talking on the phone, how long can you stay with the conversation before becoming tired, defocused, uninterested, or absent? Attention span indicates your time limit to complete a task (See the chapter "Attention Span"). Notice when you "check out."

Relapse

The time period between improvement periods during recovery is called the relapse or refueling time. Properly understood, relapse time is as valuable as improvement time. Self-esteem issues, complicated by depression, may take you off track temporarily, initiate an emotional downward spiral, or attack the ego part of you that wants to "get well right now." Relapse, reframed as refueling time, can be a strong and quiet friend (See the chapter "Relapse").

You can prevent the agony of refueling time by mastering your available energy, once you know what that is. By paying attention to your body, you can learn to prevent overextending your energy. Journaling will assist you in tracking your relapse episodes. You will be able to observe the increasing lengths of time between these occurrences and track your "integration of gain" progress. (See the chapter "Journaling.")

Word Finding

The distance between the word you want to say and your lips can extend over the horizon. Finding the word you want and speaking it in a reasonable length of time constitutes word finding. Sometimes, in that search, two words that you want to speak may come out as one attached word. These things happen. (See "aphasia" in the index.)

Part of the challenge of word finding is giving yourself permission to blurt out a word so that you can fix it. Just saying it will also help you discover the interesting channel your brain is using for words right now. Describing the word you want, by category, the language of your hands, sound-alikes, or the context of the word will also help you carve a path to it.

It is also OK to not get the word you want. Let it be. Most likely, it will show up in a few minutes. It's like any other part of life when standing in line is involved. Anxiety clearly interferes with word retrieval. Just say, "Oh, what is the word I want?" Take a deep breath, relax, and let it come. You may be surprised at how thoughtful and careful you will appear to others. (For more help with "Word Finding," see the chapter "Talking and Thinking.")

Sorting: (Part One)

There are two kinds of sorting to examine. The first is the ability to separate truth from projection. One of the interesting things the brain may do with you is to provide you with embellishments or projections within the context of a story or its outcome. You may find yourself innocently expanding upon the truth. You may find yourself telling a whopper. Your brain may not be able to tell the difference between reality and an enhanced version of the truth. Within this expanded version of the self, and the self-seeking need for the world to be OK, the brain will lower its guard in favor of more important duties. Generally, libel or perjury are not on the agenda, but colorful or more courageous renditions of reality make spontaneous appearances. Your brain is too tired to initiate a self-correction of the rendition.

It can be embarrassing to be confronted by these wonderfully exciting stories. And it would be great if the stories were true. The brain, in its search for stimulation, has inadvertently entertained itself. And sent the bill to you! (See "The Beard Butcher of Boulder.")

Sorting: (Part Two)

The second part of the sorting process deals with how your brain decides what is available to you and what is not, and when it is available to you and when it is not. Some pieces of an event may be available to you, whereas other pieces may not. It is as if part of your memory is in one storage box and part in another; one box was opened, and the other box put away, somewhere.

THIS JOURNAL ENTRY, JANUARY 31, 1992, SHEDS LIGHT ON THE EXPERIENCE.

Misplacing information or feeling like the answer is fighting its way through thick membrane curtains just to get out? If someone would just fill in the blanks, you'd remember. As if the news travels easily in through the membrane but self-generation or finding it in the Rolodex is a tremendous effort.

"Hi! How are you? It's been a while. What have you been doing?" (While all along your mind is searching frantically for the person's name, a clue, a hint, anything that will jog you to recognition. Please just tell me your name. I hurt my head and I can't remember just now.)

You know you know them. They were just put in a back closet, less important than healing the brain. It's in there, just further away than usual. Painful to not remember. Sad. My body prioritized without consulting me. Boxes of knowledge packed up and stored, arbitrarily it seems. Almost frivolously. Why can I remember how to can peaches but not remember how to put on eye shadow?

Why do I mix and jumble words, sentences, and thoughts but remember the words to Handel's Messiah and sing along with it, for five hours? Why do I ski more cautiously, protect myself in elevators from being bumped, but slide down the banister at work?

Random is how it feels. Illogical. But of course, to my brain, most logical. It feels out of my hands.

(You will learn more about sorting in the chapter "Talking and Thinking." The chapter "Retrain Your Brain" will offer specific therapy to improve your brain's ability to sort and retrieve information in a helpful way.)

Discernment and Details

The subtle decisions in life are handled through the ability to discern small differences. Discernment is the ability to be tactful, or to speak tastefully. Discernment is keeping one's social behavior on a fine line. To hug, kiss, shake hands, or tip one's hat at any given meeting is a decision made with a discerning consideration. Discernment is appropriateness at a refined, subtle level.

The details of life on the nonsocial level are a part of this discernment ability. Wearing gold earrings with a silver necklace misses a wardrobe detail one learns early, similar in nature to wearing white socks with a dark suit; it is an aspect of subtle functioning that gets short-circuited with brain injury. I found this piece of my wardrobe experience most frustrating.

THIS JOURNAL ENTRY, NOVEMBER 17, 1992, SHARES THAT FEELING.

The good news is we're working on subtleties now. Minutia. The slivers. The specks.

The bad news is I really was good at details. Slivers and specks. The struggle to recapture them is painful. For my ego. Big E. Little go, Oh, Oh. The old voice plays on. The gold standard tarnished again. Rescuing me from my ego is quite the job.

My inflated memory of my former self follows me around like Salieri (masked and caped) beneath Mozart's window, craning for just one, just one glimpse at the music through Wolfie's eyes. Just once, for old time's sake. Can't I just have it back for a moment?

Who knows which pieces I will get back yet? (And which I had best bless and be forgotten, come to think of it.) I wasn't exactly a pretty picture all the time. There were edges of unattractive behavior. Will the worst of it come back to haunt me and strike out unexpectedly like the arm replaced in surgery, donated by a homicidal maniac?

Will the minutia return, to allow me multiple mental activities once again? Or will I use sticky notes so often that stock in the company is a wise idea? Time will tell. Yet, shall ego rule? Or does my heart have some say in the matter?

(See the chapter "Lifestyle Changes and Challenges" for help with discernment and details. Also see the chapter "Inhibition and Appropriateness.")

Sequencing

Performing tasks in a logical, productive order or progression involves a continuity of events. Simple, logical events that you may have performed in a certain order for decades, such as making breakfast or getting ready for work or school, may now be, at best, impossible, frustrating, and exhausting. Following a recipe, reading a map, or even reading the instructions at the car wash may now be overwhelming, confusing, and maddening.

Along with speed and accuracy, order is very important to brain function. When the brain's wires are scrambled, the sequence of an event may slip through your fingers even when you have all the pieces of the wire maze before you.

There is a part in your brain that keeps track of what you are doing. It is a built-in monitor, checking in at regular intervals to make sure you are on task with the necessary steps to carry out your behavior. When that monitoring system becomes short-circuited, you may still know the steps and even be able to tell someone else what they are. You may not, however, be able to actually follow through on your own. Repetition, outside monitoring for cues from others, and note cards may help.

For 18 months after my accident, I was unable to add numbers in my head. I had to write everything down. My pocket calculator seemed too complicated. For someone who once was able to fill a grocery cart and know the total within 50 cents before tax, this was a sorely missed skill. I still get tears in my eyes remembering the day I could add again. I was helping out at a convention booth, selling T-shirts and mugs for an Avalanche Safety conference, when.....

JOURNAL ENTRY OCTOBER 4, 1992

Today I was able to add single columns of numbers without having to struggle or write it down and check it. The doubt seemed to have lifted. I just went ahead and added two T-shirts and a mug together and came up with the answer. And it felt good. Notation of the return of another skill. A sigh of relief and on to the next sale!

A small improvement; another piece of the puzzle; a piece of myself returned to me—long gone, found, and back in place once more. It seems a small enough issue. Small pieces are all that seem left now; tiny parts, slivers of me, prickles on my skin like walking through thistles and trying to wash the stings off. Phantom stings, illusive yet painful enough. I know they're still there. Little stings, fading but not fading fast enough. Fading, stinging, itching, scratching. Emotional Calamine, self-esteem lotion to soothe the spirit.

A painful wait; enough reward to endure the time, but painful nonetheless.

(You will find additional information on sequencing in the chapter "Retrain Your Brain.")

Follow-Through

The task at the other end of sequencing is following-through. Taking an event all the way through to completion, and also just sticking with a task, requires focus, attention span, and logical progression. It also demands stamina, as does holding the picture of the desired result in mind. Resist the psycho-babble that suggests you might not be committed, loyal, or a team player. Follow-through involves a number of executive functions working together. Your commitment will miraculously return when you can follow what is going on around you. Give yourself time.

It took me two and a half years to be able to return to the gym on a regular, unescorted, and unsupervised basis. It wasn't commitment, discipline, or desire. Not resistance nor stubbornness. Then, one day, I could do it. A developmental curtain lifted, and I finally had enough in the "follow-through bank" to be able to workout again. The overwhelm of the lights, the noisy environment, the clang of the free weights, the incessant eye contact from the other athletes, the background music, and the television white noise were gone. Apparently my filtering system finally had enough stamina to work more efficiently. I could spend my energy on exercise rather than environmental filtering. Finally!

Multi-Track Thinking and Differentiation

Doing more than one thing at a time, thinking more than one thought at a time, or juggling several different thoughts or activities simultaneously generally describes adult thinking. This ability allows us to make decisions quickly, solve complex problems or puzzles, organize effectively, and handle numerous details simultaneously. Multi-track thinking allows us to sustain and keep pace with our complex lives.

Multi-track thinking can be compared to using a computer software program such as Windows. Normally, you can open a number of windows, one over the other or in different parts of the screen, and run a program in each part. After a brain injury, you may be able to operate only one window at a time and on a limited time basis. You will have to build back up to more windows over time.

A brain injury reduces brain efficiency, causing us to be able to do only one thing at a time. When more than one thing happens at the same time, we can become lost or confused, unable to proceed or prioritize our response. We lose track of thoughts. We can neither differentiate nor focus on the issues at hand. The brain shuts off and thinking grinds to a halt. It is a helpless, frustrating feeling.

THIS JOURNAL ENTRY, NOVEMBER 17, 1992, OFFERS INSIGHT INTO THIS LACK OF ABILITY TO FOCUS.

> I feel like a mental agoraphobic. I can't get my brain to come outside. Internal paralysis. New ideas frustrate me to tears. I can only perform one task at a time. Don't interrupt me when I'm thinking. Don't change your mind after you've asked me to do something. The cruelest joke is teasing me when I'm concentrating. My mind becomes helpless and ceases. I lose both activities. I hate me and I hate you. Self-esteem and relationships take a downward turn. Then the self-loathing of recovery steps in. The spiral supports no one. I take steps to protect myself and I cry behind my eyes. For me. For you. For us.
>
> As I waited for the humor to return, I wait for this, too: differentiation. Subtle skills of concentration, determination, and sorting.

The sequence of events and their relative importance, and my ability to choose and to act.

Emotions play a significant role in brain-injury recovery. Emotional responses to cognitive frustration take thinking efforts astray. Feelings take energy, your most valuable commodity when healing. See the chapters "Emotions" and "Depression." The chapter "Retrain Your Brain" will help with multi-track thinking and differentiation.

Summary

This overview chapter on "Executive Function" defined the central terms regarding the jobs the brain performs that produce awareness and the ability of humans to carry out lifestyle activities and responsibilities. There is an enormous amount of information in this chapter because it lays the groundwork for so many other chapters. The issues raised are treated more extensively throughout the book. Other referenced chapters direct the reader to further discussion and assistance. Please consult the index for quick access, and know that the themes addressed here will be repeated and reviewed frequently to ensure that you grasp them.

14

Attention Span and Overwhelm

Your mind wanders successfully for hours, moments, or just long enough to protect you from your immediate environment. Your friends say they will call you back later, when you can talk more. Reading the comics takes an entire morning's worth of energy.

The world seems too big to comprehend as it descends upon you. Your mind is occupied by something, then hours go by unaccounted for. Life is so distracting. Your brain is overwhelmed.

JANUARY 23, 1993: ATTENTION SPAN

Is it hard to read this book? Short attention span? Affected eyesight? Depressed? Lost hope? Therapized out? Sick of being poked and prodded and still seeing no change. Group therapy full of whiners stuck in the past? One more kindly suggestion from anyone and you'll scream? One more person says, "Oh, that's easy," as a preface to your request for help on a task that used to be easy, and you're ready to punch out some lights?

The emotions around attention span can be volatile. Loss of one's ability to pay attention is aggravating at best. Yet, here you are. This is what it looks like and here are some clues for how to get through it.

JOURNAL ENTRY DECEMBER 16, 1992: OVERWHELM

There are days when being overwhelmed and failure look curiously similar. Have I mentioned the ski patrol? The volunteer branch. A wonderful organization filled with the usual good-hearted people in a nonprofit, volunteer group. Dedication, commitment, drive, overtime, and the occasional egocentric.

My last five years have been filled with sound learning, experiential outings, lots of patrol duty time, and hours and hours of volunteered time. Then I got promoted. To a regional position of responsibility.

Of course, at the same time, being overwhelmed at work (why not change careers) and at home (why not get engaged) and at play (why not become an avalanche instructor, a mountaineering instructor, and a first-aid instructor trainer) conveniently coincide.

Is it overwhelm or is it failure? Failure to what? Cope with overwhelm? Is overwhelm—or was it ever meant to be—coped with? Is overwhelm not in and of itself a containerized loose cannon? Are you feeling overwhelmed?

And where does burn-out figure into the equation? Is burn-out a function of overwhelm or vice versa? By failing to recognize burn-out, is feeling overwhelmed the next logical (?) step?

Is midlife crisis a simple label for the inability of the burnt-out mind to sift out the unnecessary chaff of life, thus encumbering the midlifer with a tidal wave of issues/events/choices indistinguishable, the water from the fishes? And time ticking in the ear as the wave approaches, leaving only ducking into the wave, hanging 10 on the crest, or mangling ashore the options open in any split second?

Is midlife crisis avoided wholesale by the simple utterance of "no" more often than one might have in earlier life? Is being overwhelmed a simple lack of discernment fueled by delusions of immortality? Do we grasp at more brass rings than we have fingers as a hedge against imagined gloom just ahead?

And, then destructively and regrettably, do we see anything less than full-scale triumph as failure? That, somehow, he who dies with the most titles wins? Top this off with brain-injury recovery, and we have the makings of a real set-up for distress. Not just failure.

I feel broken. Will I ever recover? I used to be able to handle stress. Why can't I do it now? Not the rational discussion of the relative merits of stress and life quality. Not whether or not this is all reasonable, or gentle, or humanly possible or healthy.

The injury catapults it right out of the pack onto a surreal-istic field of failure due to broken parts; no spare parts available. Not just crisis, but despair at recovery. A double whammy that shatters the self-esteem and returns one to the early days of recovery. To the time of dull mind and not knowing what questions to ask.

The hurt is somehow deeper, inflated by memory, expec-tation, dreams, desires, and hopes. No matter that the lens is distorted. The horizon, the future, is forever flawed. You don't know how, or why, or when; you just know the future is flawed.

Then, months or years later, the overwhelm or burn-out hits, and you don't just have your garden variety crisis like everyone else who buys a sports car or stops wearing high heels one day.

You get flashbacks of your flawed horizon. A hawk without tail feathers has a more graceful crash pattern than you. Today I am 43, overwhelmed, burnt-out, broken, flawed, and crashing. So I picked up the phone and resigned from two activities and cried for half an hour, mourning my brokenness.

Without a bump on my head, I might have felt a twinge of regret, a moment of let-down, a resolve to stay on top of what makes me happy and what brings me joy. The added lens brings another level of challenge to my horizon.

Author's note: Overwhelm is a verb, yet occasionally I also use it as a noun. Overwhelm is an aptly named condition and commonly used in brain-injury circles.

Filtering

While healing, the brain struggles to offer you enough energy to be able to tell the difference between events in your life. Sometimes you may be "tuned in" and sometimes you may be "tuned out." Take a first step and begin to rec-ognize when you are tuned in and when you are tuned out. This skill helps you decide whether or not you can function in the moment.

Just knowing whether or not you are present will enable you to obtain full value for your presence. It will also spare you self-criticism when you try to be here and you can't. I know this sounds like the classic oxymoron, but pay attention to when you are here and when you are absent. You will be surprised that you can discern when you are not present.

Though not true for everyone, for me, it was as if a little voice on my shoulder were communicating with me when I was defocused. I could watch the world from behind a gauze curtain but could not reach the world or influence it in that moment. The good news was that I was never in any danger any time I was defocused. There seems to be a fail-safe system built in that snaps me back in focus if impending danger (opening the oven to get the cookies out) approaches. Like a back-up battery for emergencies. This is good to acknowledge yet not take advantage of.

It is important to remember to only engage in risky behavior (driving, filling the bathtub, operating a sewing machine) after your "tuning-in" times are lengthened and after you have awareness of your tuning-out times and can stop a risky behavior, like chopping vegetables, should you tune out.

Background Noise

Living is a noisy proposition. With brain injury, the perceived volume of noise suddenly magnifies tremendously. It goes beyond loud to confusing cacophony. It gets this way because our filtering system has shut down. Environmental clamor ensues and becomes an unbearable, painful, and debilitating experience.

Formerly simple sounds like the radio, stereo, traffic, crowds, running water, television, a fly in the room, someone else talking on the telephone, food sizzling on the stove, a barking dog, or children playing outside will now all inundate your senses and overload you. Background noise is exhausting. It will sap all your energy and make your whole body ache.

Peaceful surroundings are ideal for recovery. Minimize your environmental sounds as much as possible. This may mean that you wear earplugs, ear muffs, or filtering ear plugs (for info see www.brainlash.com) that reduce background noise or sound levels. Experiment with your living area and create a peaceful, quiet space.

Ear Plugs

I love ear plugs! There are spongy ones that occlude all noise and let you sleep. There are ear plugs that soften background noise and allow important sounds in. There are soft, conforming devices that are barely visible externally.

I use ear plugs to sleep on airplanes, to take a nap in a noisy place, to give myself an auditory break, and just for some peace and quiet. Eliminating auditory input can give your brain a rest. And it can relax your face and may soften a headache, too.

Of course, never mix ear plugs and the operation of vehicles or when your full attention to detail is necessary. (See www.brainlash.com for ear plugs).

Focus

Staying on task, and even the ability to keep your task foremost in your mind, provides challenge.

APRIL 20, 1993

> Remembering two tasks has become a problem again. Going to the basement to get something, I take along something else from the top of the stairs that needs to go down. I put that item away, go back upstairs, forgetting my initial task.
>
> Once again upstairs, I retrace my steps to remember my original mission. I make another trip downstairs to complete the initial task. Grrrrr."

Concentration

Your ability to keep your mind on one task may be complicated by "wandering" as your attention is pulled elsewhere. Your ability to follow through on a thought, action, or job may be weakened. It may be difficult for you to follow conversation or to understand what is being said to you or others. Following conversation may be further complicated by background noise or the presence of more than one other person engaged in the conversation. Conversation during a meeting or general discussion may be totally outside your present comprehensive ability.

Reading may be affected as well. Re-reading may be necessary to grasp the idea. You may find yourself using a Hi-Lighter to emphasize key ideas in your reading. Taking notes may also help. Also keep in mind that your ability to read may be linked to your vision, and behavioral optometry or vision therapy may be key to improving comprehension as well as acuity.

Switching from one task to another may pose an additional challenge. Gaining focus on the second task takes new energy. Returning to the original task may take another spurt of energy. Stick with and complete one task at a time. Multi-task activities may be very taxing or overwhelming at first. Discover how to make tasks smaller and more manageable. (See the chapter "Sequencing.")

There may be times when your environment flies by without you. Jokes, long stories, or examples will escape you. These are all concentration issues and will tend to improve with time and rest.

Overload

When your brain takes in all it can handle at any particular moment, it reaches a limit and will shut down. You may feel as if your mind has drawn a blank. Although this is frustrating and scary at first, it happens all the time. Your brain has slowed its processing ability in order to facilitate healing. Your disk is full, so to speak. There is no more room in your brain right now.

You remember Dorothy and the Wizard of Oz? Dorothy and her friends get to the front gate of the Emerald City. They knock. A guard comes to the window and turns them away. We're closed, come back tomorrow, he says. The window slams shut. No debate.

That's pretty much what happens to your brain power when overload occurs. Your cognitive capacity is used up for the moment. Come back later.

Sometimes you have to take a nap or just "be," as this journal entry suggests:

MAY 12, 1992

> The depression now comes as a surprise, a feeling of wanting to hide, to go sit in front of the TV and let the electrical entertainment create a hiding space. A space of nonaccountability, a risk-free hide-out, a place of quiet, a place of no demand. I can't make mistakes in front of the TV. No one will tell, no one *can* tell. It's a refuge. Interestingly, I find myself defocused in front of the tube. Certainly it isn't the content of the programming but the space it provides that is the essence of the moment. There are times when I need to un-be or, rather, to be exquisitely in time. My sole (soul?) purpose is to be.

Can it be OK to just be? Producing nothing, in the Western sense. Or is this mental exhaustion? Am I being or am I stalled out? Am I lucky that I can sit and just be during this part of the healing?

Sometimes I feel adrift. My thinking takes leaps, contains silent moments when input is barred. I can see that you are talking to me but your message isn't making it to the blackboard. Overload is an interesting place.

I used to be embarrassed by the overload times. Not living up to my old vision/version of myself. Those moments of disengagement, swimming in words, treading water with the din of the waterfall filling my ears—block the intelligible sounds in *and* out.

Swimming in the rushing river, trying to keep my feet downstream to fend off boulders. Survival, not cognition, is the name of the game. There are moments of pure survival. Split seconds of terror. Glimpses of the void, and gratitude for the clarity when it returns.

It's not obvious to me. It used to be when I first came home from the hospital and stared off into space or lost track of conversation. In the anemia period. But once I was back skiing and driving, the *really obvious* behaviors gave way to the more subtle, refined omissions.

Those above-average areas. Where the only therapy is time. And for which the therapists had neither sympathy nor a treatment plan for recovery. What was I complaining about? I have more left than most folks ever started with. I didn't lose enough to show up on the graph. I notice it; they don't.

The Grocery Store

If you are looking for the ultimate in overwhelming visual and auditory stimulation, the grocery store is the place for you. The first Saturday of the month is your best bet to blow all available circuits.

Only the finest in bright lights, shiny floors, crowds, infants, music, noise, crashing carts, paging for a wet clean-up in aisle 3, extra staff, and shoppers in a hurry with two carts full can complete the experience.

There are times when I still cannot enter or remain in the grocery store or discount store. I have walked out of more stores because the environment so overstimulated me that I could only cry. Many a strange dinner menu has followed a quick exit from the grocery store.

I never regretted leaving a building or room that short-circuited my brain. The fluorescent lights alone can jumble vision, create blind spots, and keep the brain from registering anything worth remembering.

Just walk out. Or seek refuge in the grocery store bathroom for a while. Spare yourself the agony. If you desperately need something, go home and call the grocery store. They will deliver it. Yes, prescriptions. Yes, videos, too. Anything you want. Stores are in business to sell you stuff and will do whatever they can to make you happy. Or their competitor will. Ask for help.

Before embarking on a grocery store adventure, remember to wear a brimmed hat and sunglasses. It reduces the glare from the lights and the floors. It really helps.

Traffic Noise

The amount of activity simultaneously occurring on the highway, not to mention all the potential options inside the car, pose an opportunity to overwhelm you while driving a car, motorcycle, truck, or bicycle.

The same is true of parties, large meetings, the movies, the wind, rain, barking dogs, and other groups of noise makers. You are not required to get used to any of it. Remove yourself from any situation that overloads you. Do not sacrifice your energy or mental health. It is never bad manners to protect yourself from harm. Anyone who does not understand—tough. This is about your healing process. Take care of yourself.

Use me as an excuse, if you like. Just say, "My coach says I have to go now." Make up anything you like and blame me. Do what it takes to take care of yourself. I'm on your team.

Feeling overwhelmed is exhausting. It may take a few days to recover from a particularly overwhelming episode. Parties and idle chit chat are never worth three days in bed.

Attention process training is a systematic method of presenting stimuli to the brain to process for longer periods of time and at faster speeds. Sometimes the brain, following accidents, has a "slow rise time" or a difficult time starting to process information. Auditory overload may also cause the brain to shut off. But the brain can be trained to process information even with distracters like background noise.[3]

Brain wave or alpha wave therapy, also known as electroencephalographic (EEG) biofeedback or EEG neurotherapy, is a relatively new therapy method to improve the brain's ability to normalize brain-wave states. In fact, it may still be considered experimental by some therapists and insurance companies.

Many people with brain injuries produce an abundance of theta waves, the state of the brain just before we fall asleep. That same injured brain may make fewer beta waves, the brain waves that offer a focused and attentive brain function.

With EEG biofeedback (like physical biofeedback, only for the brain), an individual is able to see brainwave patterns on a visual screen. Given exercises for the mind, the brain-injured person can learn to alter these states and thereby possibly improve concentration. Once the individual knows what it feels like to be in these different states, she can voluntarily re-create the desired state of mind.

A research project using EEG therapy found that application of this treatment method showed the following encouraging results for the participants involved.

> First there was an increase in energy, followed by a decrease in depression or temper, then to a decrease in sensitivity to sound and light, to increased attention span, to reduction of dizziness, to vascular headaches disappearing, to increased libido, to less reversal of letters or words, and lastly, to an increase in short-term memory.[4]

Neurofeedback is a newer technology, similar to biofeedback, and is very effective. Many approaches exist, so consult your cognitive therapist for the modalities that are most appropriate for you.

Nintendo offers a product called Nintendo DG Lite, a small, hand-held game monitor into which various activities can be installed. (I recommend the white one, as that case color is the easiest on the eyes.) This product gives you a portable therapy device that will allow you to build brain flexibility at your convenience. I am enjoying games such as the "Brain Age" series and "Big Brain Academy," available at video game stores and online. The tasks are fun, easy, and designed to stimulate different areas of your brain to build cognitive stamina. Check with your therapist for additional game recommendations to supplement your brain-recovery therapy. There are also web sites that offer free or low-fee cognitive programs. (See "Resources.")

Summary

This chapter discussed attention span, overwhelm, and useful coping mechanisms to deal with these issues. The key to dealing with being overwhelmed is to reduce an overstimulating event or task to its nonoverwhelming elements, then proceed.

Diagnostic Note: There are some similarities in diagnostic symptoms between mild brain injury and either attention-deficit/hyperactive disorder (ADHD) or attention deficit disorder (ADD). If you suspect that you had ADHD or ADD before your injury, please bring that to the attention of your healthcare provider. Diagnostically, these symptoms can mimic executive function issues.

15

Talking and Thinking

This chapter discusses your brain's processing speed. Plainly, how well do your brain and your mouth work together. Coping skills and activities will be suggested to help you remember what you know and how to put it back to work.

Processing Speed

The speed at which your brain and mouth work together successfully is the processing speed of your brain. This speed will tend to improve over time as you regain energy. Meanwhile, you may experience what feels like memory loss, aphasia, word-finding disruption, and lost sense of humor.

Memory Loss

"I know that I know this. Why can't I just say it?" It feels like your memory is gone. You reach for a name, a date, or an idea, and your hand comes back empty. And you know you know it.

Could be that your memory is just fine. Most likely you are just having difficulty retrieving information from storage because of a less-efficient processing ability. Distraction from your environment or your own internal thoughts may also keep you from filtering and retrieving.

For a while yet, you may not be able to conjure up your friends' names. You may forget an appointment. You may forget where you are going in the car or why you went into another room. The word you seek may not come out or it may be the wrong word.

Cue Yourself Back

The office manager exercise in the chapter "Retrain Your Brain" will assist you in accessing information that you truly know. The "Orienteering Exercise" will also be helpful. It will demonstrate that there is more than one available path to retrieving what you know. It will show you how to access new brain cells to get where you want to go.

Aphasia

When you think one word and another one comes out, that is aphasia. When you think several words, and a manufactured word comes out, that is also aphasia. Word making is one of the most intriguing glitches of brain injury. When I paid attention to the words I was making, I got an insight into my brain's process. It helped me understand where crossed wires were and led me back to proper word making and efficient speech.

This journal entry shares my feelings about the tango danced by brain and lips.

JANUARY 24, 1993

Giving credit where credit is due: Credit the series "Deep Space Nine" for reminding me that I misused words. In this episode, the crew comes down with a virus that tampers with the brain and the afflicted cannot speak words that make sense to the listener. Sound familiar?

For me it was word making for the most part. Thought and lips out of sync. Syllables missing. Remaining syllables jammed together to make new words, like a hiccup. The intention and the result ending up in different counties.

That, or not being able to say the word itself, like a power failure in the delivery system. Or word searching, for simple words you know you know. Or professional words you paid good money to learn. And have to send the clerk back to the files to relocate. And the clerk takes his time. And you feel dumb while you wait. It's a helpless feeling, trying to remember, retrieve, relocate, recognize what used to roll off your lips straight from God's heart. Now you need a metal detector to find the filing cabinet. Wondering if it couldn't be easier somehow. Learning all this stuff the first time was effort enough. I often wondered at my career options in those days. Perhaps a nice quiet, anonymous mail-order business.

The struggle to get words out can be emotionally painful, not only for you, but for the people around you who are used to your advanced thinking. They will be tempted to give you a hand. As this journal entry suggests, you have to take charge of this one.

JANUARY 28, 1994: MY FRIENDS LOVE ME

But I couldn't let them finish my sentences for me. Or give me the words I reached for. It began innocently enough. People who love you and know you well can give you all the words you need. They know the way you think and will do it automatically. Just say "no."

Re-establish those grooves yourself! Reach. Struggle. Grasp. Work it back out to the surface. Stutter. Blank out. Use your hands. Say the wrong thing. Oh, well. Keep trying. But ask your friends to love you enough to let you work at it. That will eliminate *most* of it. That's enough. Give yourself a break too!

So the next time you want to say two words and it comes out as a one-word stew, take a breath and stretch them into the two words they want to be. Take your time. The pause gives your brain an opportunity to process.

Resist the temptation to allow your family to finish your sentences or to think for you. Although it may be convenient at the time or reduce stress for either you or for them, ***resist the temptation***. This sort of "help" keeps you from remembering what you know. It keeps you from your healing process.

Go for the mistakes. Finish your sentences, find the words you want or words that are close to what you want. You are building bridges back to the grooves in your brain that are there. If someone looks at you funny, just ask him what you said. After you are told, and you both burst out laughing, correct yourself, and move on.

Word Finding

In some cases, you may be unable to bring forward certain kinds of words. Perhaps you have a block for nouns or just verbs or maybe pronouns. Notice what is easy to say and what gives you difficulty. This can help you focus on what requires practice.

Synonyms, antonyms, homonyms, and rhymes are important. You may find some easier to produce than others. Analogies will help you rediscover your abilities with these word searches. The important thing is to pay attention to what you can and cannot do and focus your work.

Cognitive therapists are important in this area because they have workbooks and computer programs that help with retraining. You may stumble at first. Stumbling just confirms you are on the right track.

Use a Thesaurus

A little pocket thesaurus will really help when you are looking for a synonym or antonym and you need it fast. Instead of getting stuck, get help. This magic book (and its computer counterpart) helped me write this book. It's a tool. Use it.

Write It by Hand

There is tremendous value in writing by hand, using a pen or pencil, with the paper across your lap or across your desk. These diagrams will show you how to obtain the greatest advantage, brain wise, from your efforts.

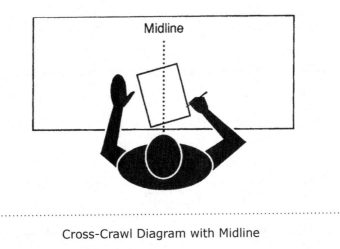

Cross-Crawl Diagram with Midline

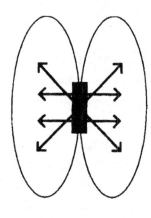

Corpus Callosum: Communication Between Brain Hemispheres

Write Instead of Type

Writing by hand makes your mind cross-crawl. It makes your brain work in ways that benefit it more than typing. Writing by hand reinforces what you know by way of physical movement, by making a kinesthetic (physical) connection among your hand, your body, and your mind. This whole-body experience of writing reconnects knowledge that you carry in your head, so that you can use it again.

Cross-crawling is a way to move your body in order to reestablish hookups in your brain from the right side to the left side and vice versa. This very simple concept improves your brain function. By crossing the midline of your body, your brain actually reestablishes connections in the process. The diagram shows, roughly, how it works.

Any activity that accomplishes crossing the midline will aid in the reestablishment of cognitive efficiency. Playing with an abacus is an example. Weaving is an example. Crossing right hand to left knee, then left hand to right knee is an example. Cross-crawling can also be done in your imagination. (See "Visualizations" and "The Phone Company Exercise" in the chapter "Retrain Your Brain.")

Clues

When I was a kid, I loved to play the game of Clue. It was fun, demanding, intricate, and adventurous, and, as a matter of fact, all of the information was there to solve the mystery. My challenge was to figure out how the clues worked together to solve the mystery.

I decided, after much thrashing about and little pieces of evidence, that I had not lost my memory (or my mind) and that what I knew, all the data I had paid tuition to learn, all the knowledge accumulated over the years, had to be in my brain still. I decided, for the sake of argument, that the filing cabinets in my brain were still full of everything I had put into them.

I decided that what I needed to do was learn how to get to those files. Early on in my recovery, as seen in this journal entry, I knew the wires were loose. This is how it felt.

JANUARY 23, 1992

There's a part of me that I miss. That I don't want to give up, but that seems to have filtered through my fingers like confetti. That piece of me that was so useful. So fun. So much a part of my expression.

Waiting for the quick wit to return. OK, sometimes it's there, leaping at the humor, painting a paradoxical scene, noticing a quirk. But, from the inside it feels slow; the speech seems garbled, stuttering, and awkward. I have so seldom experienced awkwardness. Speaking, listening, analyzing, and noticing, then responding cognitively, have always been my strong points. Recently, even graceful and wise.

And it doesn't feel gone so much as hindered. Blocked by missing wires, connectors. Stumbling over the words that emerge in no particular order. Or emerging words that belong elsewhere, as if pushed down the pipe in front of the intended ones.

Oh, how my heart aches for that edge to heal and return. To feel smooth and graceful again. To glide so easily through the thoughts and their appropriate oral transfer.

There is this part of me that seems lost. And the feeling of un-wholeness hangs like one earring whose mate has been mislaid. And if I could just retrace my steps, I feel certain that I could find it. Those earrings were a gift.

The next question was, "Where are the clues?" and secondly, "What are the clues?" Answer: Clues are everywhere. Clues can be anything. Clues are also specific to you. Surrounding yourself with what appears to be familiar, or with people and evidence that "must be familiar," is the perfect place to start.

My son had brought his new wife with him to visit us. After a few days, he asked me why I hadn't told her little stories about him. The anguish of not being able to remember events in my son's life was devastating. I couldn't recall any stories to tell. My heart was in tears.

Now, I would have asked him to retell the stories to me, to trigger my memory. The value of **external stimulation** is immeasurable. External stimulation, or external modeling, is the process of accessing or triggering your memory with the application of outside clues.

Look through an old photo album, and notice whom and what you remember in each picture. Play the "Oh, yes, I remember this" game. Look at the same photo album a week later and notice how many more faces you recognize the second time through.

Do the same with slides or photos you have taken of a trip or vacation adventure. Later, when you can enjoy a few friends over, let them fill in more blanks by showing the slide show again. Each time you view the slides or photos, more memories will return.

External stimulation can be practiced by searching through your closets, drawers, jewelry box, tie rack, kitchen, garage, and basement. Explore your environment for clues. Review your collection of Halloween costumes. Scan your book collection and magazine stacks. Rent videos of movies you have seen. View comedies and drama. Violent films can contribute to a sense of feeling overwhelmed. Viewing the cartoons of my childhood, such as Rocky and Bullwinkle, was particularly helpful. Surround yourself with clues. They provide a pathway back to your filed memory.

Your Personal Office Manager

Memory is filed away. OK, then, if memory is filed away, where is that? Files are kept in an office. Offices have office managers. I must have an office manager in my head. I must have someone who organizes and files information for me. Somewhere. I don't have to find the files. I just have to find the office manager. He can look it up for me.

This visualization of having an office manager in my head helped me formulate an exercise for requesting and obtaining information. With this picture in my imagination of a person who knew where things were, I could then ask for what I wanted.

At first, the office manager was lazy, resistant, and highly disorganized. Files were everywhere. A mess. But my systematic insistence on order, and my repeated demands for information I knew (or suspected I knew), eventually brought forth data.

Although not all information will be revealed in this way, it is one track to follow. Cueing yourself, offering yourself external clues, will surround you with your life data and trigger familiarity with your former self. There are paths back to what you know. Follow the clues. (See the chapter "Retrain Your Brain" for the "Office Manager Exercise.")

Deblocking

This may sound incredibly simplistic, and too easy to be true, but one way to unblock some pathways is to invite what you know back into your life. Practice this "re-inviting exercise" while relaxing in a quiet place. With your eyes closed and your breathing relaxed, ask your brain to acknowledge what you know visually, kinesthetically, auditorily, by smell and taste, and by intuition. Simply ask for open avenues of communication to be revealed whenever the brain is ready.

This simple request comes without pressure or stress. It is easy to understand. It is clear. Furthermore, it is in alignment with the purpose of the healing brain. Repeated practice of this technique, over time, will produce expanded results.

Sense of Humor

Some brain functions are more complicated or subtle than others. Sense of humor, sexual response, and trigonometry are examples of higher-level brain function. They are also examples of nonsurvival skills. When the brain is overloaded, these skills, and abilities like them, are not "funded."

Look to the chapters "Humor" and "Sexual Response" to learn more about how to regain your functionality in those areas. As for trigonometry, you're on your own.

Multi-track Thinking

Before brain injury, the ability to handle several activities simultaneously was a part of normal brain processing. One could perform several different skills at once. Talking on the phone, cooking breakfast, putting on earrings, and loading the dishwasher, all while watching the clock, is a common scenario of multi-track thinking. Driving a car, talking on the phone, taking notes, consulting one's Day Timer, and munching on fries is another.

Your healing brain still stumbles at prioritizing. If you answer the phone during breakfast, get ready for soggy cereal and cold coffee. Multi-tasking (different kinds of jobs at once) and multi-threading (many tasks related to a single job) are graduate-level skills. You're still in third grade. Relax, stay in touch with your inner child, and keep life simple.

Summary

The exercises listed in this chapter and others throughout the book will help you restore the skill of multi-track thinking. Talking and thinking are skills we need but skills that are hampered by brain injury. This chapter discussed various components of talking and thinking and offered some activities to strengthen those skills.

16

Sequencing

There is a certain order to life. Conducting our lives in order gives meaning and power to our actions. Having the kiss at a wedding before the vows and ring exchange would just seem illogical or out of order. Putting gas in the car before taking a trip seems right. Turning on the oven to heat it up while you prepare the recipe makes sense.

Brain injury can scramble your experiences just enough to remove you from the logical loop of progression. Steps are missed in a recipe. Turns missed while following a map. Appointments forgotten. What shirt goes with what suit and tie?

This chapter points out how the process of progression works and offers strategies for remembering what follows.

Order Is Good

In the creation of an activity, the order in which steps are taken will determine the success and efficiency of the activity. Many activities contain numerous steps to completion. When steps are forgotten or misplaced, the success and efficiency of the task are limited.

When an activity is interrupted by a misplaced step, frustration becomes the paramount outcome. Before the brain injury, the order followed for an activity may have been so obvious or automatic that you were not even aware of "taking steps."

Now your brain stops you at each step and asks for input and confirmation. What used to be obvious is now a major roadblock. You may not know what your brain is waiting for. This can drive you nuts. It feels like your brain is wasting your time.

It Takes Good Timing

Some activities require timing as well as organized steps. This is especially true of driving a car. It is good to know where you are headed and when the proper turn is required.

The same is true of cooking. Making the cake batter is a great accomplishment. Remembering to preheat the oven before beginning the batter is paramount to success. Putting cake batter in a cold oven reduces your success rate and alters your anticipated completion time.

Get Linear

Follow directions explicitly. Read all the directions in advance, and doing so out loud is very helpful. Follow the directions. (Warning: not everyone writes directions well. Cookbooks aren't perfect. For questions about the directions, ask a friend to read them with you.) Be alert to assumed steps and missing steps or instructions.

One Step at a Time

Keep your full attention upon the focused direction of the job. Involve yourself with one task at a time. Looking ahead will only slow you down and may add confusion. Do your tasks in order, one step at a time.

Get Small

Turn your task into as many small steps as possible. Each little job becomes possible when it is defined and manageable. When you can handle a small job, then you can become successful and productive. It may take you hours, even days to complete a complicated task. Just do one small piece at a time.

Take the Laundry, for Instance

Doing the laundry is a great example to demonstrate. By the time you discover that you have laundry to do, it will probably be a huge mountain.

Start with a simple sorting task. (Get several laundry baskets, cardboard boxes, or "piles" labeled with a sign.)

Begin by removing all the towels from the mountain. That will make the mountain smaller very quickly. It feels like progress! Now, sort the towels into two groups: light and dark.

○   Next, sort out the "whites," usually T-shirts, underwear, and sheets.

○   Now sort out the jeans and heavy-duty dark clothes.

○   Now sort out the "colored" clothes, usually casual wear. What you have left is usually "delicates," or dry-cleaning. Make a pile of items to be dry-cleaned and put it by the front door. (Add the "dry-cleaner" to your errand list.)

○   Now, wash a load of towels. Then hang them up or put them in the dryer. Fold them and put them away.

○   You have succeeded in sorting out the laundry and organizing it, and have completed a load. Do one load every day, and you will soon be caught up.

Driving Across Town Doing Errands

You already know that you have to go to the dry-cleaner. You may also have to go to the grocery store, the gas station, the post office, and the book store. Draw a map of these five destinations.

Make a list of the order of importance of your errands. (If you get tired, you may want to bail out of the activity. Make sure the most vital errands are noted.)

If it were me, I would go to the gas station first, since I probably need gas to complete the errands. The grocery store is important. (Could you have them deliver?) The dry-cleaner is important. (Do they offer a free pick-up service?) The post office is important. (Could you buy stamps by mail, or have someone else mail that package?) The book store is important. (Is their inventory available online? Can you mail-order?)

So, buying gas is very important. Everything else, in the event you run out of energy, can be handled differently, or on another day.

Make your route map in the order of the importance of the errands to you. You may find that you can complete all of your errands. ***That's great.*** You may also discover that you have other options.

Have the map and list of errands in your car. Using a clipboard will assist you with keeping control of your map and list on the seat next to you. Take a pen and scratch off each errand as it is completed. Trace your progress on your map so that you know where you are.

When you arrive home, congratulate yourself for completing your errands. Make a new list of remaining errands. Remember to add a new item to your errand list: the date to pick up the dry-cleaning you just dropped off!

Following a Recipe

When cooking, follow the recipe. Read it through completely. Make a list of all the things you need—pots, pans, spoons, measuring cups—making sure you have all the ingredients on hand. Lay it all out. Preheat the oven. Make sure you understand all the words and techniques that are requested. When everything is in front of you, begin. (Don't answer the phone.)

Putting on Make-Up

With the help of a friend, assemble your make-up kit. On an index card, write down the order of application, destination, and product name with color of each make-up item. Keep the card with the products. Follow the instructions on the card, and successfully create your personal look. (Declutter your supply and toss out old products.)

No Job too Small

If the task you are performing is still causing you frustration, break it down into even smaller pieces, until it is comfortable. No task can be in too many small pieces. Your creativity will emerge as you chop jobs up into workable pieces. The smaller the piece, the more confidence you develop as you complete it. The more confidence, the more success.

Soon, your brain will begin to link tasks and remember how to sequence. This may be slow in coming, since sequencing is a complicated function. That's OK. Just keep plugging away, one task at a time.

Just like skiing, you practice making a turn. Then another turn. Then another turn. One day, you can make all three turns without stopping. Another triumph in sequencing (and a good excuse to go skiing, if you need one).

Listening to Directions

You are walking down the street. You stop someone and ask for directions. She says, "Oh, that's easy. You go down there three blocks, turn right, look for the red tulips, go across the street and up the staircase by the black sign."

You thank her, and still have no idea where to go. Your mind is blank.

First of all, when someone tells me "Oh, that's easy," my mind immediately turns off. I go straight to my low self-esteem place and know that it will not be easy. People don't mean to hurt my fragile feelings, but if I knew how to do something, I wouldn't have asked in the first place. I know it's easy. But I still can't do it. Not today.

After I got over that piece of my experience, I began to ask people to write their directions down. If they persisted in saying that it was easy, I would inform or remind them that I was having trouble keeping everything in my brain, and I really needed it to be written down.

Then I took control of the problem, and began to carry pen and paper everywhere I went. When I asked for directions, I would write them down. Then, no matter how "easy" it was, I could figure it out. That technique got me to more places with less emotional damage. Excellent idea.

Sorting Your Mail

Even a task like opening the mail can seem daunting. Before you know it, the pile on the dining room table is so high as to be impossible to deal with. In the meantime, your unpaid bills mount up, you miss out on reading your birthday card from your favorite aunt, and the credit cards in your wallet have expired.

I devised a simple method of sorting mail. Make three piles out of what you receive.

○   Pile #1—Personal mail from real people whom you know

○   Pile #2—Bills from companies you recognize

○   Pile #3—Junk mail

Pile #1: This is the pleasure mail. Read at your leisure.

Pile #2: This is responsibility mail. Put it in your bill drawer and deal with it once or twice a month when you pay your bills.

Pile #3: Throw out all solicitations and advertising. Feel through the envelopes of the remaining mail for enclosed credit cards. Open those envelopes to search for cards that you ordered. Shred unwanted credit cards and throw out everything else.

Consider owning a paper shredder. Shred any paper garbage that contains personal information about you, such as your address or a random account number. Shred unsolicited credit-card applications.

A Product from Heaven

After three years of lists, calendars, and sticky notes I finally discovered the Franklin Day Planner. There are lots of day planners on the market, and this one works exceptionally well. It is easy to use, it holds everything you need in one place, and it comes in all budget ranges and sizes.

Call the company's customer service number, 1-800-983-1776 Monday through Saturday, 24 hours, or visit their web site at www.franklincovey.com. They will send you a catalog, which includes the address of the store nearest you. Their service representatives are courteous, helpful, and attentive. They will help you tailor your Day Planner to fit your daily and professional needs. They offer classes to teach you how to use the system. They also offer video classroom and audio tapes. The ***Franklin Day Planner*** will help you stay sequenced in your life activities.

For the last 16 years, I have organized my personal, professional, and volunteer life on the pages of this product.

Cell Phones

Hang up and drive. For a person recovering from a brain injury, multiple tasks are stressful and overwhelming. Operating a vehicle, paying attention to traffic, and chatting on the phone do not mix. Pull over to talk.

Summary

I quit wearing eye shadow because I could not remember where the blue went and where the purple went. While that is probably a good thing,

I now know that different strategies could have allowed me to keep my daily regimen more intact.

Sequencing accepts external modeling to remind it what to do. (See the section "External Modalities.") Break down your activity into little jobs that are possible. Experience success in many small measures. Sequencing will come back. And all the tasks that require sequencing will return with it. Humor, joke telling, storytelling, following directions, following recipes, carrying on a detailed conversation, and being able to do things like writing a book will return to your repertoire more quickly with your encouragement and support.

I was able to write this book because I chopped it up into lots of tiny jobs. Different systems work for different people and for different tasks. Write in your journal how you broke down a job into its successful components. When a task bogs you down, perhaps your journal will remind you how to enact the procedure again. Your journal is a record of your healing progress as well as a resident coach.

Remember, when you can't determine or recognize the next step in a task, ask for help. Everyone has trouble gaining perspective on the task they are knee-deep in. Where was I?

17

Stamina, Fatigue, and Energy

Recovery from your injuries is a long lasting, time-consuming, and exhausting experience. Your brain keeps you quiet and inactive. Any effort to exceed the set boundaries results in fatigue. Sometimes seemingly inconsequential behaviors like getting breakfast or taking a shower can bring on the need to rest or nap.

This chapter discusses why you get tired so fast and how to use rest, pacing, and timed tasks to effectively build and utilize your stamina.

ENERGY: Think of the energy you have as if it were a pie. This pie is normally divided into sections according to use. There is Emotional Energy, Cognitive Energy, Physical Energy, and Energy Reserve.

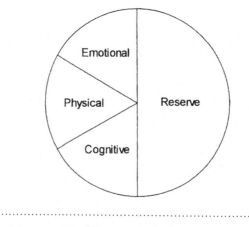

Normal Energy Pie. (Copyright: Mary Lou Acimovic, MA.)

Types of Energy

Emotional energy is generally used to suppress negative thought processes, to modulate emotional responses, and to put the brakes on unproductive reactions. When this system is overloaded, emotional energy experiences irritability, frustration, anxiety, a short fuse, quick tears, and mood swings. Depression may be triggered, setting in quickly or taking its time. You will have no reserve to defend against depression.

Cognitive energy is generally used to comprehend, filter (80% of the brain's energy is used to filter information, mostly in ways that we don't notice consciously), organize, formulate, plan, remember, monitor and validate responses, and provide you with a sense of time and place (orientation). When this system is overloaded, the brain works more slowly and less efficiently and becomes disorganized. The filtering process decreases and mental confusion may ensue.

Physical energy is generally enrolled to maintain posture, to reduce muscle tension, to move you about, to fight off illness, to program motor responses, and to inhibit and direct motor activity. It also offers you a sense of your true energy level. When this system is overloaded, you may experience fatigue, pain, decreased immunity, and headache, among other symptoms.

Reserve provides you with additional energy support when needed. It lets you know when you engage it and lets you know when it is about to run out. It is there to enhance your energy expenditures when necessary and otherwise sits quietly by.

Reserve is generally not readily available following brain injury. You push and nothing pushes back. Or you push, getting something, and then you pay for it with days of exhaustion. You may not be able to tell when to stop pushing. Therefore, pacing yourself is essential, even when you think you are feeling well. Never take reserve energy for granted again.

When any of your systems have exceeded their capacity to perform, life will become overwhelming. Those systems that perform automatically, such as your physical energy, are at risk. Emotional modulation is, however, the most fragile. Overload will offer inconsistent energy, providing you with good days and bad days. Until you understand how to cope with and manage your energy use, your life will seem out of control and out of your hands. It is.

Being Tired

When you get to the end of your energy before you get to the end of your day, you get tired. Culturally, getting tired is very uncool. Looking like you are tired makes you a candidate for jokes about vitamins and more sleep. Being chronically tired turns into a label of lazy, anemic, or goldbricking. Not pretty.

Tired is what will happen to you with brain injury. The brain uses about 80% of its energy just filtering information and environmental input for you so that you can think straight under normal conditions. When light, sound, movement, and environmental noise are not being filtered, you are an instant candidate for stimulus overload. When you least expect it, your energy pack will cut out and you will be out of gas. This experience is not negotiable with your brain.

Fatigue

Running out of gas is exactly the feeling one gets. Especially if you add a deserted highway, the middle of the night, and no gas can to the scenario. Oh yes, no money either. Fatigue feels like being stranded. Trying to function in the face of fatigue is grueling.

JANUARY 25, 1993. FATIGUE: RUNNING OUT OF GAS.

Brain-sourced fatigue can strike at any time. Pressing on is painful and unproductive. When your mind says "I have to leave (get out of here—stop doing this—stop thinking—I'm overwhelmed—I'm overloaded) now," believe it, and, no matter what Emily Post or the parents on your shoulder have to say about it, serve yourself. Leave. Because you are out of gas. And because being overwhelmed turns to frenzy, frenzy to panic, panic to tears. And you're just out of gas. Go hide. It's not your fault. Your brain has shut you down. There will be no more business transacted here today.

You've gotten enough sleep, you've eaten right, you may have even taken a walk or stretched—this isn't about being tired. This is about pernicious fatigue. The brain can only heal and work simultaneously for so long. Then, thinking shuts down in favor of healing. It will last as long as it lasts. There are no tricks for getting a few more miles out of an empty tank. You are closed. Nurture yourself. It could be this way for several years. And fatigue may strike at any time.

Pacing helps. When I first went back to the office, I went for half a day and took naps between clients. Then, over a year, I worked up to two half days and so on until I was up to three days a week. Then I tried four days a week, my original pace, and found I couldn't do it. Too much focus, too much energy required.

I wasn't the old me, but the new me. The new me could work three days a week. I decided to restructure my life to finance three days a week. Got an office partner to take my other two days, lowering my overhead from the back door.

Lowered my standard of living, paid off my credit cards, checked out videos from the library, became a coupon clipper. Sold unused household items. Had a spring garage sale. Got a third housemate. Used the pressure cooker more. Made my own pizza. Turned the furnace down and put on a sweater.

Listen to your brain, or you will find yourself stranded on the interstate for no apparent reason. You can't fight back once the fatigue has set in. Your brain will let you heal and improve as long as you *listen*.

Being a good inner listener is a key to optimal re-emergence. The clues may be subtle at first, but ignoring little clues will earn you a slam dunk "what's your name, your address, how do you get home from here?" Blank. Slam dunk.

Pacing

Once you understand that your resources may be limited, learning to pace yourself helps. The goal is to obtain balanced periods of work and rest. Balance is found when your needs are met. You may find that 10- or 15-minute stretches are what you can manage. You may find that you can work or think or talk on the phone for five or 10 minutes, then you have to rest for half an hour or more before you engage in focused thought again. Eventually you may be able to work your way up to 45 minutes on, 15 minutes off, throughout the day.

There were times early on when I could either make breakfast OR eat breakfast, but I could not do both. Eventually I paced myself so that I prepared meals that I could then eat half an hour later. I only made the mistake of pouring the milk on my cereal in advance once. Some things you never forget, even with this attention span!

Stamina

Physical stamina develops slowly, and pacing helps. I used a kitchen timer to help me keep track of time when I was engrossed in activity. Keeping track of time makes you aware of your efforts. Support yourself and stick with the pacing. And, remember, don't be fooled. Just because you feel great when the timer goes off doesn't mean there's any reserve there to back you up. If you keep going, you risk fatigue. Then you may have to regroup on your pacing and take it easy for awhile again.

Cognitive Stamina

When your brain works consistently, and you feel competent, then your brain function is operating with cognitive stamina. At first you may feel or think inconsistently. Or you may think or feel consistently, but for only 20 minutes. Eventually you will have a good brain day (see the chapter "Good Brain Day") and feel like a million bucks. Then, of course, you will likely crash and be back to pacing again. I suggest journaling that good brain day so that you remember it later when reinstating your goals.

There may be blank spaces in your continuity of thinking. Rest, exercise, and journaling can help fill in the spaces.

The effort required to build back your stamina can be exhausting, too. Small, incremental tasks will build upon one another and create a matrix of success, however small the steps. Use the same approach that occupational therapists use when returning people to work. (See index for "work hardening.") Incremental tasks, performed well, build upon one another. The length of time and length of competency increase, and soon you can sustain activity for half a day and then for a whole day.

Keep track of your progress, and watch yourself become stronger, more consistent, and more durable over time.

Talking on the Phone

A great deal of cognitive energy is involved when using the phone. You must talk, think, listen, sort, evaluate, consider, respond, and hold your attention span, simultaneously. Add to that the screening out of your environment, and a phone conversation may extract more energy than you have. Time your phone calls, and screen your phone calls with caller ID or an answering machine. Just because the phone rings, you don't have to answer it. Just because you are sitting down at home, or even in bed, the energy gets used. Pace yourself. Phone calls take their toll.

Integration of Gain

Integration of gain is a fancy phrase that describes the pattern of healing for mild brain injury. The figure below shows that the person with a mild brain injury will experience improvement times (progress), plateau times, modest loss of momentum (refueling), and then begin improvement again. Notice the steady overall gain in this model. Remember this model when you experience a bad brain day.

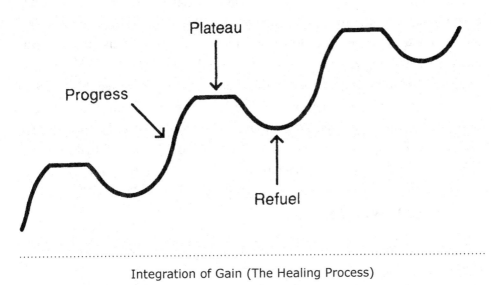

Integration of Gain (The Healing Process)

Relapse: Having a Bad Brain Day

Relapse, or discovering that you are very out of gas, happens. The more you progress and heal, the more likely you are to test your limits. The more you progress and heal, the less frequent are the relapses. Hence, there is a terrific shock value when relapse catches you off guard.

MAY 16, 1995

But I was doing so well. Now look at me, lost on the freeway, tears blocking my vision, unable to make sense of a map I've read 100 times, going to a place I've been before. I am hopelessly lost, driving in blinding snow, two hours late. Trembling, I stop to use a pay phone in an industrial area. The phone is broken.

(You may wish to consider owning a cellular phone.)

So it seems! Luckily, you have a journal. This is a good time to reread the parts about when you could not drive, could not see or think clearly, or even comb your hair. It is a great time to read or listen to the script entitled "I'm OK Today" (See the chapter "Retrain Your Brain.") See your successes. Acknowledge your progress.

Tomorrow will be better (write that down in your journal). Tomorrow will be better. Review the figure, "Integration of Gain", on the preceding page for a visual reminder of the healing path.

Even after 15 years, I still experience relapse, though less frequently. It will creep in and bring me to my knees. This happens. Now I just acknowledge that it's a bad brain day and take time to care for myself in this moment. Days like these are particularly entertaining when they are combined with ovulation, changeable weather, or the full moon. Because of these factors, I have privately suspected that there is a correlation with the menstrual cycle. When I keep up on my progesterone cream and herbs, relapse sessions seem to grow further and further apart. I suspect that the damage done to the hypothalamus during a "brainlash" keeps the rhythms of the hormones off balance (See the chapters "Relapse" and "A Good Brain Day.")

Sleep, Rest, Nap

How you used to sleep (light, medium, or log) will be different now. You may require incredible amounts of sleep, rest, and naps. Forget your judgments about napping, and pay attention. The most efficient way for your brain to recover is to make you rest. Your brain will take any chance it can get and will arm wrestle you for the remainder. And your brain will win. When your brain wants you, it will ask nicely once. Your ability to recognize this request will enhance your relationship with your brain. Your inability to recognize this request will be a losing battle and will take tremendous energy expenditure on your part if you resist.

Nap as much as you need to, yet monitor yourself so that you are sleeping through the night. If napping interferes with a good night's sleep, then adjust your napping. Some neuropsychologists suggest no more than two naps per day, of 1 to 2 hours' duration, unless a full night's sleep can be accomplished with more daytime napping.

OCTOBER 23, 1992

You may not sleep well. You may sleep like a log. At night. And any other time your brain wants you down for a nap. Opposition is fruitless. Any attempt to avoid the nap will result in mental stupefaction, loss of focus, and a tremendous force of will used up in a flash.

If your brain wants you to sleep, then sleep. It's a sign that your brain needs something. It does not signify anything about you. Not a reflection on your responsible nature, your work ethic, or the amount of time in your day to complete your artificially invented schedule of tasks. It only and simply means your brain needs you to sleep right now. So listen.

It's a lot like the dentist. If you hold still, open wide, and breathe calmly, this will be over sooner (more like the gynecologist, too, upon reflection).

Being dragged to sleep is a helpless, confusing feeling. Decades of training got you dressed and to the office. The phone is ringing, and people have an appointment to see you. You, on the other hand, are sinking fast.

Cancel the appointment and turn off the phone, lie down, and close your eyes. It may be an hour or two, or 20 minutes. It's not failure, incompetence, dereliction, or lack of "inner strength." It's a nap. Necessary after brain injury to aid the long-term recovery process. Nap now.

Holding up old pictures of yourself in your head, remembering who you used to be, trying to be her now, is very painful and destructive thinking. And it doesn't work. So just take a nap. It is as simple as that." (See the chapter "Power Nap.")

The Energy Pie

This next section presents a clear, clinical view of the use of energy by people with brain injuries. To me, this is a peek into the knowledge and notes of a cognitive rehabilitation therapist trained to help the brain injured. It is also written in clinical style.

WARNING: If this section is too clinical or hard to concentrate on, you may wish to reread it again six months from now. Ask someone in your support system to read it and to summarize it for you. The main concept here is that you only have so much energy at any given moment, and there is no reserve to draw upon. When the gas gauge reads empty, it's the truth. (*Note:* This following section is ideal reading for family members, as it summarizes and clarifies the issues of energy.)

Energy Allocation in Mild Traumatic Brain Injury

Individuals recovering from mild traumatic brain injury report remarkably similar symptoms.[5] Among these, fatigue, or lack of energy, is so consistent as to be almost diagnostic. Even individuals who perform within normal limits on standardized testing complain of overwhelming fatigue following the effort. A complicating factor is that the fatigue is often attributed to depression that leads to psychological treatment rather than consideration of the fatigue as a condition that predisposes a patient to depression.

(Diagnostic note: Strangely enough, these same mentioned symptoms are prevalent among stressed college student populations. If you were a full-time college student at the time of your brain injury, be aware that you may have had these symptoms beforehand. The brain injury could have enhanced those symptoms.)

Normally, a person is not directly aware of energy expenditure. One becomes accustomed to having adequate energy reserve, not only for routine daily activities, but also for tasks that are more energy intensive. Rarely does one exhaust the reserve. Phrases such as "at the end of my rope" are commonly used to acknowledge that one is close to running out of energy. A person knows when circumstances will be enervating that would not be disturbing if reserves were adequate.

A person who has sustained a mild brain injury is, however, frequently susceptible to overload. Practitioners who treat these clients know that "overload" is a word that transcends linguistic boundaries and is immediately identifiable by those who have not yet named their experience. I have found it useful to develop a functional explanation that allows clients with mild traumatic brain injury to put their experience in context and regain a sense of control.

The energy allocation model (referred to by clients as the Energy Pie) describes normal energy requirements in emotional, physical, and cognitive terms. Because many energy-intensive functions are taken for granted, it is helpful to point out aspects of one's daily life that do require energy or exertion.

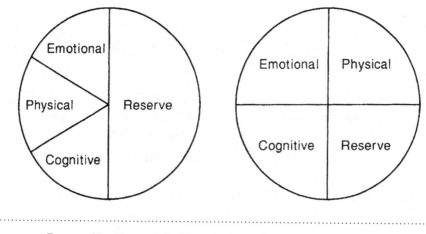

Energy Pie, Normal (left) and After Mild Brain Injury (right)

The client is alerted to the following COGNITIVE demands

(1)   Executive functioning, including organization, planning, and
       follow-through
(2)   Language function: comprehension, formulation, and
       expression
(3)   Memory: attentional aspects, storage, retrieval, incidental, and
       prospective
(4)   Monitoring and validating responses
(5)   Sense of time and place (orientation)
(6)   Filtering

This last item, filtering, is particularly important. It is obvious from
a functional standpoint that the brain must use substantial energy to filter
irrelevant information, both internal and external in origin. The process
occurs to a large extent at a subconscious level. Clients with mild brain
injury report increased susceptibility to distraction, reduced tolerance for
noise and light, and difficulty concentrating while driving. It is important for them to understand these difficulties in a context that then allows
them to manage their environment while working to improve tolerance to
distraction.

PHYSICAL energy requirements include

(1)   Maintaining posture (Because of physical injuries, clients often
       need to pay more attention to posture as they can no longer
       tolerate sloppy habits. Unfortunately, they have less energy to
       devote to this subtle attentional task.)
(2)   Reduction of muscle tension (Muscle bracing due to soft tissue
       injury is common in this population.)
(3)   Programming, directing, and inhibiting motor responses
       (Reactions are often slowed.)
(4)   Fighting off illness
(5)   Managing pain

Few clients with mild traumatic brain injury escape the pain of muscle-
tension residuals.

Our clients are surprised when we inform them that it is normal and healthy to be depressed, given their current situations.

EMOTIONAL energy is required to

(1)   Interpret negative thoughts
(2)   Formulate emotional responses
(3)   Modulate emotional reactions

It takes energy to regulate oneself emotionally when recovering from a brain injury. An emotionally "healthy" person does not expend energy warding off depression. It is important to realize that your emotional lability may be "without reason" and that, if you possessed the energy to regulate the responses, you would. This information is, unfortunately, sometimes in direct contrast to the advice of well-meaning psychologists who aggressively treat the depression as if it were a cause instead of an effect. With brain injury, you may not be able to modulate your emotional body because you simply do not have the energy to do so.

Once a client understands normal energy allocation, it is easy to use the model to demonstrate graphically why functioning is disrupted. The "normal" model shows that one can access reserve consistently, at will, depending upon the requirements of the situation. When an injury is involved, we explain that the normal reserve is tapped on a routine basis. Pain, for example, a common coexisting symptom, constantly drains available energy. Anxiety over persisting cognitive and physical symptoms is also a significant factor. Cognitive complaints ("slow thinking," difficulty concentrating, susceptibility to distraction) indicate that more energy is required to perform at pre-injury levels in terms of both quantity and quality of work. Practitioners experienced with this population are not surprised when clients report "effort headaches" ("my head feels swollen," or "my head is going to explode") following periods of concentration, indication, perhaps, of increased energy requirements for cognitive tasks.

Because more energy is required for routine daily functioning, less reserve is available for tasks that require additional energy expenditure. One will continue to access reserves when necessary; however, now there *is* a danger of exhausting resources. When this happens, overload occurs. Quite simply, the system's capacity is exceeded.

The client is helped to understand that overload can be experienced cognitively, emotionally, and/or physically. Cognitively, clients report "shut down" ("computer is down"), disorganization, confusion (e.g., getting lost or losing track of a conversation), decreased filtering, or increased distractibility. Physically, fatigue is most striking along with decreased tolerance for pain. Clients insist they are sick more often or recover more slowly. Emotional overload is experienced as increased irritability, frustration, anxiety or short fuse, crying easily and for no reason, and emotional lability (mood swings).

Once the client understands the principles of energy allocation, s/he is able to improve his/her ability to predict overload. Of course, it is not really that simple. One must also be a good self-observer and reduce symptoms of denial to function efficiently in predicting overload.

S/he can begin to assess available reserves, often in concrete physical, cognitive, or emotional terms, which allows adjustments in schedule, inclusion of necessary breaks to recharge, and reduction in duties. It is also then possible to help family and friends (as well as therapists who may impose unrealistic demands on the patient) understand the heretofore unpredictable behavior of the client, minimizing unproductive responses. Clients are often frustrated when emotional outbursts occur. When the reason is "overload," the client's response may be discounted, causing further frustration. Treatment can also focus on energy management. Clients can learn how much they are able to do in a certain amount of time based on existing resources. Gradually, they learn to reclaim control over their lives as they recover from this all-too-common and poorly understood injury.[5]

Permission to Sit and Stare

Many days I sat and stared. Too awake to nap, too tired to activate, I would sit and stare. For minutes, sometimes hours, at a time, my mind would defocus and wander off. I seemed to need that time away. I don't recall that I held thought, processed ideas, visualized, or dreamed during those times. It seemed like a wakeful rest.

In a private setting, this experience is very helpful to the healing process. Practiced at the workplace, it may be misunderstood. (Discuss this possible behavior with your workplace advocate.) Be aware that you may sit and stare. Give yourself permission to engage in this behavior. As far as I can tell, it is beneficial in a quiet place. (Obviously, it is not wise if you are driving a car.) Sit and stare all you want. Enjoy this form of rest as you gain energy in your healing process.

Brain Bucks

The unit of measure I devised for quantifying how much energy an activity cost me is called *Brain Bucks*. This imaginary energy currency helped me define the comparative expense of my exertions. For instance, a pre-injury visit to the grocery store cost 100 brain bucks; a post-injury visit to the grocery store cost 3000 brain bucks. A pre-injury car drive across town during rush hour cost 300 brain bucks; the post-injury car drive across town during rush hour cost 4000 brain bucks.

Use the brain bucks system to evaluate the level of stress that any activity has upon your system. By assigning numbers, the brain bucks gauge determines what it will take. You can quickly ascertain your fee and, therefore, your willingness to pay the price. Using the brain bucks system helps you decide if the activity is worth it or not. It's your money.

Summary

You are your energy pie. Awareness of your energy situation will explain a great deal about your behavior to yourself and others. You only have so much energy, and you do not know how much there is at any given moment. When you feel like you are running out of gas, you are. Believe it and act accordingly.

18

Risk and Initiation

Are you holding back, dropping out, declining invitations? Is your fear factor increasing? Does fear of failure keep you from proceeding and serve to remind you that you feel broken? Are you hiding in the safety of your house? What does it take to get you involved?

Risk and initiation are two vital elements of executive function. They are prime symptoms of mild brain injury and tend to show up after physical injuries have subsided. Just the thought of going back to work or school can cause anxiety, deepen existing depression, and compound mental processes. This chapter explores the aspects of what you may have come to perceive as an unsafe world. We will examine the reality of the fear and the courage of taking risks.

Agoraphobia

Agoraphobia is the term that describes the fear you feel that, when leaving the safety of your house, you will automatically be placed in harm's way. Are you hiding in your house? Have your pets, plants, TV, stereo, and newspaper become your trusted companions? Is there a lot of sitting and staring going on? How about a lot of sitting and crying? Worn anything but your bathrobe lately? Do you often wonder, or care, where the week went? Welcome to the club. Your brain has successfully encapsulated you in the safety of your home. That is your brain's job.

You are OK. This situation is temporary and will lift as your healing process continues.

The Unsafe World

Your brain knows that you cannot think fast enough to protect yourself from harm. So, for your own good, you may perceive that the world is a scary, fast, dangerous place and that you may not be able to protect yourself. This thought will lift gradually as your brain becomes more proficient with processing abilities.

You are OK. And the world is no more safe or unsafe than it was before your injury. You will regain a more balanced view of your environment as your healing process continues.

Sitting and Staring

Sitting around doing a lot of staring off into space will be a big part of your lifestyle for now. Forget everything you ever thought about sitting and staring. It is now good for you.

This journal entry will shed some light on the subject:

JANUARY 24, 1993: INITIATION AND RISK

Your brain quiets you to protect you. When you were hurt, your brain assumed a new job: the preservation of the host. With a survival instinct of brutal compassion, the brain enrobes you and enrolls you to keep itself alive. And since your last significant input to the brain was trauma, you are under house arrest until further notice. The brain accomplishes this with depression, lowered self-esteem, lowered physical activity with possible weight gain, no enthusiasm, no ups or downs, no risk, no danger, no fun, no interest, no attention span, no extreme emotions, not much of anything. Nothing new is allowed. New thoughts, new directions, new occupations, anything anyone could cook up to raise your spirits/income/self-esteem/fun or activity level is verboten.

Sitting around being unmotivated is exactly what suits your healing brain, and it will do everything in its power to get that result.

Crying? Staring off into space? Watching lots of mindless TV? Driving and can't remember where you are? Reading every part of the paper but the "help wanted?" Can't pick up that phone to get a hair appointment? Sitting and staring at your exercise bike? Waiting for the mailman is your goal for the day? Putting off taking a shower all day? That's your brain at work, doing its best to protect you. Remember your "worst-case-scenario" thoughts? Like someone swerves in traffic and your mind finishes the story complete with dead bodies and 911 responders from 40 minutes away? I even put a pair of latex gloves in my car in case I was at the scene of one of these accidents (before I got my HIV test results back from the blood transfusion I had received).

Finally, I was able to purge these thought chains from the mind, slowly at first. Close my eyes fast and say "no." And think "that is not real." The worst-case scenarios still come, but they are less traumatic, and I send them packing as quickly as I realize they have their little talons in me.

And all this time, your brain is operating with good intention to keep you alive as long as possible. A noble cause, no doubt. But dismal prospects for fun, expansion, adventure, and risk. Especially in the face of rehabilitation, which involves at least expansion and risk.

Your force of will has only so much gas on any particular day. Making consistent activity difficult. Especially when fatigue (mental, emotional, physical, and spiritual) becomes a predominant player. Your "old" brain is running the show. Your willpower operates consciously, and only by your focused effort, not much chance of overruling the old brain when it's traumatized. The house makes the rules and owns the bank. Your purse is empty and there's no credit for desperadoes in these parts. Much obliged if you'd take your business elsewhere.

Wait a minute, you shout back, I pay the mortgage around here, what's the big idea? The old brain waves a power of attorney under your nose, with your birth date on it. You were just a baby then, that was so long ago. Surely it isn't still legal.

Plenty legal, old brain says. And for your own good. You're lucky I'm here to take care of you.

But I'm better now, I have to move on, support myself, learn how to live again, figure out who I am, what I can do and how I'm going to live.

I'll be the judge of that. You're in no shape to make decisions. Go sit down. Relax. Clear your mind. Better yet, take a nap.

You clench your fists as you grow sleepy, staring straight ahead, thinking of nothing, doing nothing, wondering little, moving less, dehydration sets in, your appetite wanes, you forget what happened. Even the summer cloudburst outside gains only your passing interest.

Maybe tomorrow I will try again. Or the next day. Soon, anyway. *This can't last.*

Hesitation

What is your risk profile? When do you hesitate and why? Quite likely you are hesitating constantly or frequently. Quite likely you will resist opportunities that are familiar to you or that you have accepted in the past.

The mental frustration is not only exhausting, but embarrassing as well. The logical brain says, "I know how to do this." The healing brain says, "Too dangerous, too complicated, too soon." The logical brain counters with "But I do this all the time." The healing brain glares back with "Too tiring, too slow, too much."

Along with hesitation, risk, and initiation comes the outcome: ***beginning again***. In the course of recovery, you will begin again and again. You will start over a lot. This is OK.

These two journal entries focus on hesitation and beginning again.

APRIL 14, 1993.

> Taking risks, or rather following my personal bliss, has added another layer of challenge. Pulled between things I have been good at (organization, politics, activism), and things I'm being pulled toward (weaving, writing, publishing, ministry), and might be good at if only I weren't intimidated by security (mortgage) and new ideas (brain injured).
>
> I didn't used to be slowed down by something as silly as finances. I'd have come up with six ways to figure the budget another direction and five ways to write them off. But ever since the "fall," I've been looking over my shoulder at the checkbook, watching carefully each month. Constant stress. Wondering if my receivables will show up in time.

Risk Taking. Initiation. Writing. Panic.

APRIL 15, 1993: INITIATION BE HANGED.

> I recently dreamt that my life was changing and I'd have to start all over again. The feeling of dread and exhaustion (and the

unusual feature of the dream being in black and white—I always dream in color) (I can hear you dream analysts buzzing out there) and the "here we go again" thoughts carried me into a somber morning.

Which "begin again" was it? The rebirther/immortalist "you must be willing to begin again" jargon? The soup is burnt so toss it out and "begin again?" The baby with the bath water? More college? New house? New state? Or new attitude?

Is this a black and white issue? Or am I a new person now, different by a twist of circumstance? Can I love the new me enough to quit making her live up to my old memories? Can I create new ones? Can I just proceed?

May I begin again for the very first time? Am I starting over or simply starting? Which is the more gentle path? Would it be easier to check my ego at the door and get on with life? Not old, not new, not borrowed, not blue?

Just life? No suitcases, file cabinets, or scrapbooks of who I should be, could be, or would have been. Rather, who I shall, can, and will be and, in fact, am right now. (You self-esteem buffs are eating up this part.)

Quoting Popeye, or God, or Goddess, whomever you prefer: "I am what I am" or "I am that I am." The "I am." The self. The power of self-proclamation, of beingness (beingness is such an "in" psychobabble word—forgive me).

Understanding and claiming the self. A process, a passage through childhood (you early childhood development types help me out here), repeated during midlife crisis for the faint of mortality.

Suddenly, then not so suddenly, the brain-injured person must find her way back to self, in an adult body, looking perfectly OK at the office. To discover, explore, claim, test, and claim again for the first time her identity, her essence, her self.

To search out—without benefit of adolescence, a safe haven, or parental support—her identity, her place, her name. To carve, mold, and shape in a few months or years (if the mortgage holds out that long) what her progeny have 10 to 20 years to explore, taste, and experience.

The logical mind chants "get a job" as if ShaNaNa were in her living room, while her intuitive side searches for a fit, gropes at options, and scratches the surface of lead after lead, frantic for a sign, a revelation, a bolt of lightning, or even a trickle of light on the path. Looking for home.

Home for the soul. A place to be that rests the spirit and feeds the mind and body. Vacation. And not just what shall I do, but what can I do?

A sense of panic floods over me. The clock ticks louder every day, reinforcing not only the lateness of the hour, but also the poignant lack of progress that looms larger every day.

What can I be? Who can I be? Where can I go from here? The approach that broadens and narrows simultaneously. Wanting to open up. Fear of being too slow. Believing that the door of opportunity slams shut according to Murphy's Law.

Doom and destiny, my nighttime companions as the green nightlight slowly turns from a 3 to a 4 and I lie not sleeping, reminded by yet another automated techno-gadget that marks my stalemate. Universal coordinated time.

So here I am, starting over. Not from the beginning assuredly, but certainly newly started. And vocationally altered. Not to mention avocationally. The search for the self. A quest or formal development? Both perhaps. No lark. No light reading here. For me, a serious task of reclaiming/claiming my course. Just a firm thump on the compass to free the needle and allow me to be on my way.

On my way, with all the awkwardness of an adolescent with none of the benefits or protections. A gangly, disjointed adult. A kid in a business suit. A minister with zits. Waking up one morning and none of my "shoes" fit. Held to an external standard my inner eyes cannot see. Trapped in my body, wishing to free my mind.

The Jump Start

Some days there is the irresistible urge to think that, if you could only get a jump start, you could get going again.

MAY 25, 1992

So, why am I still sitting here? Wanting to watch TV. Yearning for someone/something to drag me off hiking or camping or biking. I used to go everywhere. Alone, with others, no difference. Now I sit like a slug and stare off in space.

Even with my new love interest, I have to dig deeply to get motivated. The world is my oyster, and I'm turning the platter away. My mind seems less internally sourced than before. Less creative. Less alive. Less vital.

I must remember (I keep telling myself) that the recovery could take two years. And I'm only halfway finished. Yes, I will keep getting better. Just keep getting up and trying again. As many times as it takes. As many times as you have to ask for help. When you look just fine. Especially when you look just fine. Just keep getting up.

The Bootstrap Lecture

The jump start is your internal wish to get on with it. The Bootstrap Lecture is what you get from people who don't understand your experience. Because you look fine, there are people out there, the rugged individuals, who think you should be able to "get over it," "get with it," and "get on with it." These people are clueless.

The truth is, if you could have reached your bootstraps, you would have pulled yourself up by now. But your brain has cleverly hidden your bootstraps for your own good. The "American Bootstrap Method" of self-extrication applies to people with stamina, focus, and determination. You don't have those ingredients at the moment, and your brain, which is busy getting better, is not going to return them to you.

So, do not listen to the Bootstrap Lecture. It does not apply to you. You might wish it did, but it doesn't.

Vulnerability

One of the clever ways we protect ourselves both emotionally and physically is to attempt to disappear. When feelings of vulnerability arise, becoming smaller and quieter seems like a good idea. We may find ourselves dressing blandly, speaking softly, or not speaking unless spoken to. Raising a hand in a meeting is unthinkable. Walking in or out of a room full of people is avoided. Raising one's voice becomes impossible.

Becoming invisible is certainly one way to succumb to the pressures of perceived vulnerability. Notice if you are doing anything along those lines, and gently remind yourself that you are temporarily perceiving the world differently than you used to. You are OK. This will pass with time.

Keep breathing, and limit any unnecessary information in your world that reminds you of danger. (Television news, newspapers, violent videos, movies, cartoons, and some music and video games are general sources of visual danger.)

Why You Are OK

Your enthusiasm for life, your self-esteem, and your personal safety are linked together. Having fun may seem impossible right now. Risk seems gigantic and overwhelming right now. That first step may paralyze you today or even tomorrow. But one day soon that curtain shall rise.

Before my accident, I was an adventurous hiker, mountaineer, rock climber, and backcountry skier. Glaciers, mountains, and treetops were my playground. All that stopped suddenly, and I was a lioness on the couch for six months, caged in by blankets.

Remember by Performing Familiar Skills

One day I thought I was ready to remember. It occurred to me that, if I tried to do things I used to know how to do, I might remember how to do them again. The theory was that I would regain confidence by remembering what I knew. This seemed logical. So my boyfriend took me glacier climbing in Rocky Mountain National Park.

We hiked in several miles, carrying an ice ax, crampons, daypack, and lunch. We reached the foot of the glacier and decided to climb straight up to the saddle of Hallett Peak.

JULY 4, 1992: THE FOURTH OF JULY.

Put the events of those days together. Days filled with being out-side rediscovering myself in nature. Three that stand out in recent memory include the stranding on Mt. Rainier (my successful self-descent to Camp Schurman) and the summer hike in Caribou that allowed a special freedom of the hills to be restored to me.

And this third, a most excellent Saturday afternoon in Rocky Mountain National Park, an afternoon that began early morning, dawn's pink glow on Long's Peak, up before the campers even rolled over in wakeful dreams of deer and squirrel. On the trail, up and up, headed for Tyndall Glacier, miles ahead over boulder fields and snow patches too small to stop for crampons.

Boulders, snow, sun, wind, rock, dirt, flowers, water, spider wells: The trick is to gently pick your way through, leaving the spiders undisturbed in their quest for food. Walk around the flowers. Tread lightly here. The thriving is pricey in this neighborhood.

Up to the glacier, strapping on the crampons, remembering the sequence, cranking them on. They are my claws for the face of the glacier.

We choose a line below a small cornice and begin to move up, easily walking, then "au canard" (the polite French term for walk like a duck), then the angle increases and we begin to kick steps. Plant the ax, kick feet, plant and kick, up the high angle face, 800 feet, two toe pockets at a time. Straight up, the cornice crowning the exit to the saddle. Dan tries to mount the cornice, but the slight overhang prevents the route. We traverse right, where snow meets rock, secure to the face with metal toes and an ax dug deep. A slip here takes one swiftly and not so gently to the and the boulders below. Focus on the task is paramount.

Mixed climbing means gripping boulders with metal claws on your boots. The exit from the glacier requires a few steps on snow, a few steps on rock, then snow and a place to sit and remove the claws once (safely?) on the saddle. So, right about 12,000 feet on the edge of the cornice that crowns the glacier, we look at our watch, then the weather, then the summit of Hallett Peak just 1/2 mile and another 700 feet away. Lunch at the summit!

I start out, the wind whipping my skin, following the cairns that appear quite suddenly and peacefully in a reasonable line toward the summit, through a smooth saddle of granite slabs, lichen, moss, and miniature flowers reaching an inch or so toward the sky. That's when I hear "Stay" spoken by my left ear. I turn toward the voice to see a panorama to the north as beautiful as it always has been for thousands of years. But the speaker has ridden on the wind and is gone.

Higher up the mountain, in among the final boulders that grace so many summits in the Rockies, the speaker returns, to my right ear this time, and says among the winds, "Whisper." I do not look about this time, for the trail requires my full attention and the view to the south holds its own spectacular moment once I reach the top.

We dine upon sandwiches and rice crackers, enjoy a map and compass problem, then begin the journey home.

If you walk straight up a glacier, how do you get down? The fast and scary way, of course. Dress in waterproof clothes, sit down on the snow, and nudge yourself over the edge, even if you can't see the destination below. *Not!*

Roll onto your front, in self-arrest position, and slide down with all the brakes on until the angle is friendly to a sled ride. Then flip over and ride, ax as a brake at the hip, for the journey to the bottom.

Watching for ice, rocks, and such, which may be less than an enjoyable sensation to buns. Yes, I sit up here a long time, afraid to hurl myself over the edge, over the lip. I sit and examine my many options, all of which look exactly alike. The longer I sit here, the wetter I become. Discomforts begin to outweigh one another. Time to go. A few calming breaths, roll into self-arrest and take off the brake.

Down I go, beginning to enjoy it, judging the slope and rolling back to a sitting position when the angle appeals to me. Then from enjoyment to delight. Then satisfaction. I did it. Like so many other skills I'd reviewed and remembered today. Remembering those little skills, techniques, rules, and cardinal rules for being in this wild and beautiful place. This wilderness of rock, snow, ice, wind, flowers, and picas. This place where our water comes from. This place that spawns both our clean air and our pure water, where nature works her magic and mystery that we may thrive at her feet. Walk gently here. Magical and sacred acts are afoot. We are guests to a gracious host. Remove your shoes at the door.

Summary

The factors inherent in risk and initiation are not generally operative for the brain-injured person during early recovery stages. Notice this, allow for it, and focus on self-esteem and the healing process during this time.

19

Inhibitions and Appropriateness

This chapter deals with the "leap-before-you-look" aspect of mild brain injury. The inhibiting factors of socially acceptable behavior and appropriate activity are impaired. Discernment, which is the brain's ability to sort out and choose acceptable conduct, diminishes with injury. Behavioral good taste takes a break.

These issues are mild, generally, and may not extend past what you might not do at the office but you might do at a New Year's Eve party. Alert your healthcare provider if your behavior becomes suspect, especially in the opinion of your family members.

This chapter will help you decide if your social judgment and behavior have been affected by your injury. It will also let you decide if this new part of you is OK (if a little eccentric) or if support, awareness, or intervention is indicated.

The Self as Loose Cargo

Brain injury may alter one's ability to sort out what is socially acceptable or appropriate. One may become too loud, too open, too insistent, too unbridled, too much fun, and certainly too honest. These can be dangerous if not embarrassing behaviors in the wrong setting or before the wrong people.

There is this welling up of emotion, without restraint, that reacts before thinking. The most painful part is that you may not know you are behaving out of context in a specific situation. You may never know, or you may realize with chagrin at a much later time.

Discernment

Discernment is the brain skill of sorting out, weighing, and balancing behavior before it is enacted. Discernment is what keeps social behavior civilized. Discernment restrains people in polite Western society from asking about another person's salary. Discernment stops one from ordering more food than one can eat. Discernment controls your wardrobe selection before going to work or to church. Discernment tells you what is right and what is wrong. Discernment inhibits unsociable or potentially criminal behavior.

Inhibition

We all know someone who could use a little "loosening up." The shy, stoic, and stern are hard to entertain. A little food, beverage, and soft light might help. Occasionally a breakthrough occurs, and the person either blames it on a spiked drink (not his fault) or adds the breakthrough experience to his lifestyle and relaxes a bit.

Increased inhibition accompanying brain injury may have no more than this effect. On the other hand, it could rock and roll.

JANUARY 18, 1992: THE EVIL TWIN

Then there's this new part of me. This part with a life of its own. This part that reaches out and acts spontaneously, almost independently. There's this new part of me more uninhibited than I was before. And I can't say I was a shy person to begin with. Sliding down the banister at work. Doing a headstand in the clinic. Skiing on sand dunes in a belly dancing costume.

So when the psychologist suggests I might be a little less inhibited, I can clearly smell trouble. He asks me if I've been acting "differently" lately. Since the banister is my baseline, I look deeper and find more. Eating salad with my fingers in a restaurant. Hollering out my car window to some unsuspecting kid on a bike to wear a helmet. Speaking up in meetings. Acting on my emotions; coming from my heart without checking in with my head. I feel louder. Less reserved. Less dignified. Bigger. Unabashed. It's uncomfortable. But more creative.

Is this who I am now? Will this part alter somehow? I'm scared. Will I say or do something to hurt or harm another and lamely plead "brain damage?" There is this self-doubt, this wondering, this hesitancy. But only in my head.

My heart's new life enjoys this freedom. Like a puppy chasing a butterfly. There is an innocence about it. And a new ease in expressing compassion.

The enfoldment of this aspect appears to carry on. I prefer not to fear but to love this part as an endearing eccentricity. As a friend who loves faster, acts quicker, speaks out, and enjoys deeply. Not bad things.

Good Taste for the Brain

Inhibition disorder can bring out the zealot in you.

FEBRUARY 13, 1993: HELMETS

Hurting my head converted me into a helmet fanatic. I don't mean that I began wearing a helmet everywhere. Actually, it meant that I began to roll down my car window and admonish bicyclists, bikers, skateboarders, in-line skaters, and anyone else within earshot to "get a helmet." Oh yes, my inhibition center was altered, too. So, warning people about the travails of brain injury seemed my duty somehow, having been there. Knowing the pain. Reaching out to spare others as best I could. A missionary from the "do as I say" school of public address.

Sadly, of course, a helmet would not have prevented my experience, having scrambled the Jell-O that was my brain against the inside of the skull. That and the oxygen deprivation from the ruptured spleen.

Yet the helmet seems a symbol nonetheless. I proved an obnoxious missionary with a heart of gold, preaching to the brain-bucket deaf. The newly uninhibited part of me knew no differently. I wanted no one to suffer and lose as I had. My message knew no shame.

I sure hope that that kid on Broadway asks Santa for the helmet. And that he gets through summer safely.

The Lumbar Brain

This is the term used at my house when an excuse for uninhibited behavior is necessary. Best to have a handy excuse.

Shopping can be a dangerous adventure. Best not to buy new clothes and to stick to your safe and sane outfits until the governors are back on duty. Good taste cannot prevail, and cleavage simply will not do at the office.

Judgment

Knowing your limits is a challenge. You may think you can do something that you truly cannot. But you can't tell the difference. Until maybe later. After it's too late, and the deed is done.

FEBRUARY 14, 1993: THE BEARD BUTCHER OF BOULDER

Sometimes that new, uninhibited part of me takes on a life of her own. Take, for instance, the length of my fiancée's beard. A bit bushy; due for a trim.

Of course, I volunteered to trim it. How hard could it be? Out came the manicure scissors and comb, and, presto, trimmed beard. After all, I have trimmed my own hair on occasion.

Well, he didn't have to shave it off, but it ended up a bit shorter than we had anticipated, shall we say. Later, he asked me if I'd ever done beard trimming before. Of course, I told the truth. No. But how hard could it be? This new part of me is certainly as long on enthusiasm as it is short on skill.

Beards, Helmets, Cleavage

This new part of yourself may be a romp or a roller coaster ride. Best get to know as much about her or him as soon as possible. There is certainly plenty to laugh about … later. Make an alliance with your loved ones that they will assist you in times of unbridled inhibition. Give them permission to quiet you down, suggest a new outfit, or remove you from a conversation headed for disaster. It may not be as much fun as having your way with the world, but it can serve as a model of appropriateness once you have recovered from disinhibition.

Limbic Rage or Having an Episode

The outer reaches of decorum may be challenged by what is called limbic rage, episodic dyscontrol syndrome, or more kindly "having an episode." It is similar in onset to a seizure because it is uncontrollable and usually begins with an aura prelude for the person who experiences it. The episodes may be misunderstood and misdiagnosed, as manic depression for instance. A limbic rage may be caused by a lack of oxygen or a brain injury that affects the limbic system.

The rage episode itself may be triggered without warning or obvious provocation. A minute change in schedule, environment, weather, diet, or music may be all it takes. The family members live in constant vigilant awareness of the possibility of the rage occurring. The affected individual lives with the fear of flying out of control at any given moment.

Generally, the rage episode can last a few minutes or up to a few hours. Different from a simple loss of temper or crabby behavior, limbic rage is irrational, primitive, and often violent in nature. During an episode of limbic rage, people may destroy the immediate environment, harm themselves, or harm anyone who tries to restrain them. The episode gives the affected individual extra physical strength, so normal restraint tactics by family members are met with primal force.

Fortunately, limbic rage comes in varying intensities. Many people maintain a shred of self control and can divert their behavior to less destructive targets.

Contributing factors to the triggering of limbic rage may include sleep deprivation; sensitivity to sugar, alcohol, or allergies; and biochemical, environmental, or hormone changes in the body. Premenstrual stress is often a major contributor to rage episodes.

Once the rage episode has subsided, the person is exhausted and may enter a sleep or nap stage of several hours. The energy consumed by the limbic rage may plunge her into a period of fuzzy thinking and nonproductivity for a few hours or up to a few days. Dehydration is also a factor, so push fluids to dilute the adrenaline during the recovery phase. Consider administering Rescue Remedy (by Bach Flowers), available in health food stores. I consider it highly valuable in restoring a sense of leveling of mood.

During it all, the loved one is horrified by her behavior and defenseless to prevent it. Self-esteem sinks immediately, and destroys self confidence.[6]

MAY 7, 1995: LIMBIC RAGE

I read the article to my husband as tears streamed down my face. With halted breath and a sense of relief at the same time, I described to him what limbic rage was. The article outlined what happens to me, usually just before my period, when I fly out of control and say really stupid things.

The article talked about the irrational behavior. It outlined the difference between limbic rage and general anger or emotional behavior. It described the "aura" state just before onset. For me, that was the "we're going to have a fight" feeling. Then the rage would begin, followed hours later by the total physical collapse, the exhaustion, and the brain shutdown.

After an episode, I was usually unable to think, speak well, or move around the house with any spark of energy at all. Fuzzy brain, closed for the day.

I looked at my husband and said, "They named it. It's not my fault. There's really something wrong with me." I was elated. Naming it made it smaller, understandable, not about me. I felt relief. Dan replied, smiling, "Lucky me."

Summary

Your good taste and sense of decorum may have taken a hike. Awareness is a good thing. Focus on loving this new part of you and on learning as much as you can. Dysfunctional discernment or disinhibition can be temporary or permanent. Increased inhibition may self-correct or linger. Limbic rage may be with you throughout your recovery. Know that you are not alone. Ask for support, pay attention, and try to stay out of trouble. Should your behavior reach past socially acceptable parameters, notify your attorney that your defense should consider limbic rage as an aspect of explanation for your behavior.

I have acquired some great Halloween costumes in the past few years. Now we're talking channeled inhibition!

Part IV

THE TOOLBOX

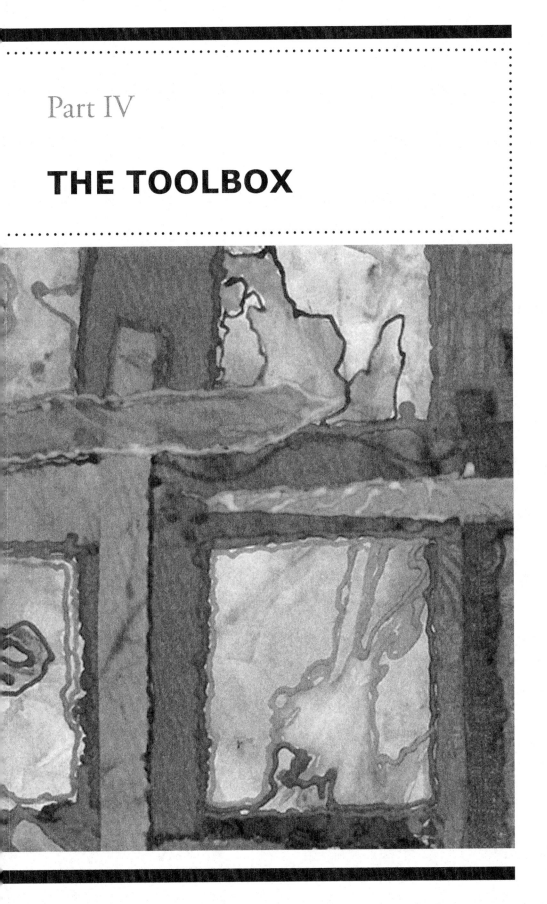

20

New Abilities and New Skills

Integrating your new abilities and new skills as they are revealed is important to your overall progress. Your brain is different now, and it is very important to discover exactly in which ways it is different. Many recovering people realize they see the world from a new point of view. In fact, brain-side preference may have switched. You have heard of left-brain people and right-brain people? The linear or technical thinkers generally access the left side of the brain for those abilities. The nonlinear or creative thinkers generally access the right side of the brain for those abilities. Although most people have a healthy balance using both sides of the brain, one side tends to dominate.

Electrical engineers who suddenly discover a talent for piano? Painters who become architects? Perhaps their brain-side preference has shifted. This chapter will discuss various aspects of discovering how your new brain works. It will also suggest ways to enhance learning and to help you develop new information pathways.

Inhibition

One of the most interesting aspects of brain injury is the change that may occur in your ability to inhibit yourself. You may be less inhibited than before. If your brain was right-brain dominant, or you have switched to more right-brain use, inhibition issues may be a new aspect of your personality.

So, just how bad can this be? Well, if you were severely inhibited to start with (never calling attention to yourself for any reason, for example, or being unable to use a public restroom unless you were alone), any move toward a more open style could be appalling, at least to you.

If you were outgoing, prank loving, joke telling, and costume wearing to begin with, you could become too loud, change your clothes anywhere, slide down the banister in a stuffy office building (this is great fun, by the way), or jubilantly interrupt someone's conversation.

In either case, a healthy sense of how to deliver a sincere apology for committed acts of disinhibition will go a long way toward smoothing out your life. It is always easier to ask for forgiveness than for permission. And since you really cannot help yourself anyway, and your motives are pure, a heartfelt apology supports everyone. (See the chapter "Inhibition.")

Holding yourself in horrified contempt, judging your actions, or punishing yourself is counterproductive. Sending yourself to your room without dessert will not accomplish the dispatch of a message to your brain. Punishment falls on deaf ears.

Your brain is different now. Finding out who you are, in the best-case scenario, is to embark on a grand exploration. Notice, appreciate, and discover the new you. Lighten up. You can choose to be gentle with yourself. Being eccentric is easier than being out of control. And eccentricity is a culturally acceptable role. You decide how you view yourself. Choose a gentle path as you explore.

Years of Training

Because I was brought up in a very practical, economical, stoic, and disciplined family, inhibitions were a part of our family training code. Certain behaviors were simply "not done." Imagine my horror, then glee, as I worked my way through the inhibition jungle.

FEBRUARY 29, 1993: BLACK UNDERWEAR!

All my years, Spanky pants or their boring woman-sized equivalent have been the rule in the top drawer of my pecan and brass dresser. Years and years, decades indeed, of sensible cotton briefs. No tacky panty lines to call attention to my anatomy. No unsightly bikini waistband cutting across the view like a sunrise horizon. Always a lighter color than the outer garment. Rules to live by.

Then, one day, feeling the need to break a mold set in steel and welded shut with mother's words, a pair of black cotton briefs (I really stepped way out on this one) found their way into my dresser. They are easy to see in the drawer, the midnight among the sea green and pastel jewels: a footprint on the pale sand.

Wearing them is another matter. In a dimly lit restroom, dressed in winter woolies, I pause to rise and, to my amazement, I cannot see my undies. Trusting that they are in place, melding with the deep blue gabardine, I grasp, stand, and gently lift all garments toward my anticipating waistline. That secure feeling returns.

(I wrote this piece while waiting for a lecture by Natalie Goldberg, author of *Writing Down the Bones*, a book for people writing a book. Having found the dimly lit restroom, my brain could not differentiate between the dark colors of the layers of my clothing. At first I was frightened, then simply trusted that, being winter, the underwear had to be there. But the trick on my mind still stung a bit, though less than a year ago. Another sign of the healing process: more laughing, less fear.)

Your Inhibition Quotient

Equation:

Your previous inhibition + your new liberation = blessing/curse.

How you solve this equation is your choice. How you view yourself in this equation will lead you on a path of comfort or torment. If this is a painful question, look at what is wrapped up in your ego. Then ask the question again and again until the pain subsides. Ultimately, this is a journey toward self-love and acceptance.

Discernment, Sorting, and Appropriateness

A faux pas is one thing. Telling the difference between appropriate and unacceptable social behavior is quite another. Discernment is the ability to grasp and comprehend what is obscure, or hard to pinpoint. It is the ability to discriminate, or to see what is not evident to the average mind. It is the power to distinguish and select what is true, appropriate, or excellent. It is the ability to have insight into a situation and to apply sympathy or understanding. It is the ability to search with the mind, employing keen practical judgment.

Wine tasting, for instance, takes discerning taste to sort the crisp from the flat, the oaky from the smoky, the California from the French.

Sorting is the ability to group similar items together. Following a conversation in a crowded room while eating snacks successfully would be a good way to know if you are sorting each activity and responding to it. Spilling the food on your tie, talking with your mouth full, or allowing your eye contact to wander would indicate that you may not be sorting sufficiently.

Sorting requires a ranking of events, items, or ideas in order of importance. Keeping things in order or "sorting things out" so they are in order and you can deal with them is vital.

If the phone is ringing, the house is on fire, you have to go to the bathroom, and your toast is ready, what do you do? If you cannot answer this question, you are not sorting for highest priority. (*Answer:* The caller will call back; you can pee next door; and you can feed the burned toast to the squirrels later. *Get out of your burning house!*)

Appropriateness

Are you compatible with your surroundings? Are you responding in harmony with the activities around you? Do your answers match the questions posed to you? Do your behaviors fit your environment?

These are not deeply emotional questions. These are simple questions. If everyone else is in semiformal dress, sipping cocktails, are you in a clown suit and Goofy shoes? Between movements at the symphony, are you the only one clapping and rising to your feet? Are you blowing your nose at the banquet table? Making amorous advances toward the clerk at the checkout counter?

Well, maybe you misread the party invitation, but the rest of this stuff is simply inappropriate behavior.

If you are aware of your inappropriateness but find yourself temporarily unable to control your behavior, practice the heartfelt apologies mentioned above. If you are unaware of your inappropriateness, enlist an advocate to assist you in navigating this labyrinth.

Switching Brain-Side Preference

For simplicity sake, let us refer to the left brain as analytic and the right brain as artistic sides. Have you noticed that you are more expressive and artistic than you were before your injury? Have you become a fix-it person or Web surfer? Are you relating to your environment differently now?

New Grooves in the Brain

We have all heard about the legion of unused brain cells in our heads. Well, now is the perfect time to access them and ask for help.

Your brain, though temporarily healing, has many untouched cells just waiting to be invited onto the team. To incorporate them effectively, it is important to pay attention to how you learn.

We all learn differently. Some of us learn auditorily, with our ears—if we hear it, we learn it. Some of us learn with our eyes—if we see it, we learn it. Some of us learn by hands-on—if we touch it and make it work, we learn it. Most of us learn with a combination of all three, with one style being dominant.

Discover for yourself which style of learning you are using now. It may or may not be the same style you employed before the injury. Once you know which avenues are most open to your present learning style, engage those approaches when learning new things.

Learning

At first, learning something new may be too energy draining. Take it slowly. You are in the process of retraining your brain to serve your new needs with the resources available. Pay attention to how you think your brain is working. Follow thought processes and patterns that you notice. Stay alert to newly revealed pathways. Your brain is different now, and, the more you learn about how it takes you from A to B, the sooner you can unlock the routes.

Life-Choice Changes

There may be choices from your old life that you remember as having been important to you. Now they seem not only unimportant, but stupid and not worth your time. You may have this reaction to ties, small talk, shaving, cocktail parties, gossip, brand-name things, the four food groups, the "team," spectator sports, the news, the newspaper, political debates, the office party, or personal hygiene. Of these, only the last is a sign of depression and requires attention. Well, the four food groups (chocolate, pizza, ice cream, and take-out) are important, too. The rest can be left behind and re-examined later, or not.

Your life is different. What you select or don't select marks the boundaries of your lifestyle.

Left-Brain Person and Being Ethically Overwhelmed

If you are an injured, left-brain, analytic person, all these changes may bring a cloud of disbelief and fear into your life. The control and order that defined your existence, your career, and your professional reputation may disappear. When this need for order and control are attached to your total identity and to your code of ethics, a difficult challenge is ahead.

Justifying and balancing the changes may be frustrating and fruitless. When this happens, talking it out with a professional therapist who understands your situation can be very valuable. Together you can forge a path that supports your ethical and professional abilities while integrating your newly found talents.

Right-Brain Person and Being Overwhelmed by Stimulation

For the artistic right-brain person, when the door opens to the analytic world, the opportunity for overstimulation is high. Additional psychic experiences or being overwhelmed by creative ideas can set in. This person has no knowledge of how to turn all this stuff off, or how to reduce or control the flow.

Dreams become too real and generally contain intense themes. These dreams can even affect your waking day with their intensity. The ability to inhibit grows weak, and the "outgoing personality from hell" may emerge. This person may find herself speaking the truth as a child would, with no sense of consequence or appropriateness. In the words of the left brainers, the right brainers go "nonlinear."

Enhancing Your Learning

The chapter "Retrain Your Brain" contains several visualization exercises that assist in reconnecting your brain and enroll unused cells to forge new pathways to barricaded information. The design on the front cover of this book is a cross-crawling "chart" that you can use to assist in reestablishing the pathways between the two sides of your brain.

The Cross-Crawling Chart on the Front of the Book

Use the front cover of this book as a tool of recovery. Set the closed book squarely in front of you, in your lap or on a table. Trace the design with the index finger of your right hand. Now reverse your pattern.

Trace the design with the index finger of your left hand. Now reverse your pattern.

Now rotate the book 45 degrees, and repeat the entire exercise. Remember to breathe deeply during the exercise, following your finger by moving your eyes, not by moving your head.

DECEMBER 31, 1993: WEAVING

Next month my weaving journey shall take me to Navajo weaving class. I feel drawn to it somehow, as if by an ancient voice seducing me down a path, returning me to something I have known in another incarnation.

The draw to this work is uncanny. As if I already know which music to hum as I sit before the warp and entwine the woolly yarns spun and dyed the previous winter. It holds a feeling of "coming home" to my soul.

Summary

For each brain-side–dominant group, the loss of control is similar and the sense of the loss is intense. Making your brain your best friend again will take time and effort on your part. Pay attention to what you notice. Journal your findings. Your therapist may be able to help you put the puzzle pieces together. You have to gather them.

Above all, remember to let go of judgment with this process.

21

Retrain Your Brain

External triggers remind you of what you know. External triggers also can be used to retrieve your knowledge base. Something as simple as going to the library can open a memory door.

This chapter will take you on many journeys of discovery and recovery. It will give you tools for tracking down information, for setting up new pathways to information you know is in there, and for using underemployed parts of the brain to rebuild your thinking power.

Read and use this chapter slowly. The temptation to overachieve exists. Remember, your brain can still reach out and slam dunk you for piling on too much work. You are still healing.

External Triggers

Go/see/feel/smell/listen/do. Let the world be your path back to your memory. External triggers, those hints and reminders of your world, are vital to brain activity and information recovery.

Seek experiences that remind you of what you know. Watch old movies. Frequent familiar places. Visit book stores, libraries, cooking shops, flower shops, video stores, museums. Go where you used to go. Picnic in a familiar place. Trigger your memory in the context of your ordinary life. It will bring back what you know you know.

It may take more than one reminder for some information to return, or for you to retain the thought. That flower, that tree, the name of the song that plays over and over in your head, the movie plot where the butler did it.

Every information stimulus will open a door somewhere in your brain that will eventually lead to something you know.

Yes, "it takes time." But you can nurture, encourage, and mentor that time back to quality recovery with enhanced self-esteem and useful tools necessary for your new life ahead.

I took a weaving class so that I could have fun while practicing sorting, sequencing, and cross-crawling. You may find an activity (new or familiar) that serves and supports your learning needs. Weaving now serves me by feeding an artistic part of me brought out by the brain injury. I blossomed in a new direction that my old analytic brain would not have originally considered. Now there's a floor loom in my living room and yarn all over the dining room table.

Listen to your inner voice when selecting a fun activity that serves your recovery needs and style. Games are important. We teach children how to learn with toys and fun games. Visit a toy store and explore the possibilities. Just remember to avoid Saturday or holiday times when the crowding and external stimulation are greater.

The layered weaving design on the front cover of this book is an artistic outgrowth of my healing process. From the initial visualization of the concept, I assembled these wondrous fibers together to form the cross-crawl pattern you see and use today.

Explore the possibilities. Venture out into your world. There is much to recall, and, while you have fun, your brain will be remembering. Stay mindful of your energy level. You may need a nap after play!

JANUARY 16, 1993

> Still not a believer but willing to try something else, I signed up for an eight-week weaving class. New words, new medium, complicated mechanical object, patterns and sequences, a proper order, a teacher who will whack your hand with a ruler if you pull the wool the wrong way (reminding me of vicious stories of terrorist penguins in the halls of secular education), and a classroom full of normal people.
>
> Got out my bifocals, chose a red pen to make visible notes in the text, selected two contrasting yarn colors for the obvious tasks ahead, and discovered that I understood the material, whipped through the lesson, and enjoyed not only the learning, but the lovely little thing I was weaving as well.

Brain Orienteering

If you have ever tried the sport of orienteering, you know that you receive a map, a compass, and locations on the map to which you must personally hike or ski. You are not limited by how you find the target locations. You just have to find them. The first person back to the starting point having found all the targets on the map "wins."

Sometimes the pathway to a piece or body of knowledge is blocked by a bruise, lesion, or scar. Plainly, the message cannot get there from here. The path from A to B is not available to you. The road is closed.

So, I was thinking (such as it is), that perhaps the orienteering premise would work for retraining the brain. I theorized that there are uncountable unemployed brain cells just hanging out, waiting for an invitation. What if there were more than one way to get from A to B? What if the unemployed brain cells could build a detour route?

The New Way to Get There from Here

What if I could ask my brain to find another pathway to a piece of information? Based on the unemployed-brain-cell theory, I began to experiment with this concept. By using hypnotherapy, and visualizing the diagram of the new pathway as shown, I created a simple tool.

Orienteering Exercise

Assume a comfortable position in a quiet and softly lit environment. Begin to relax, closing your eyes, breathing softly. Focus now on your breathing, paying attention as you inhale and exhale. If your mind wanders, just focus on your breathing. Sink deeper into your comfortable position, and enjoy the quiet of listening to your breathing for about two minutes.

Now, imagine and picture in your mind that there is a point A. Point A asks a question. The answer resides with point B. A roadblock prevents you from proceeding directly to point B. You now invite the surrounding and available brain cells to find a new route from point A to point B. The available brain cells are most happy to help you out. They find a new route to point B. You thank them.

You may find that the new route is very simple, or that it wanders all over the place before it gets to point B. That is just great. You got there, you got help doing it, and you have new members of your team who will help you again, just for the asking. When you have completed the visualization, focus on your breathing, and return to your full wakeful state when you are ready, refreshed, and peaceful.

Rest assured that, in your wakeful state, you may ask for this help again. The answer to your question may take a few minutes, hours, or days. But the answers are more likely to reveal themselves with the aid of your new team members. This also takes the pressure off you to generate data. Give it over to the available brain cells. They can handle it!

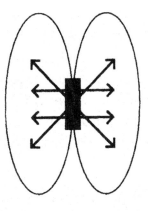

Corpus Callosum; Communication Between Brain Hemispheres

MARCH 23, 1993: GO TO THE LIBRARY

The library has always been one of my sanctuaries. A haven of knowledge and peace. A place to find out. To learn, discover, and ask.

After my fall, the library disappeared from my life. And it installed computers. The library became an overwhelming place. The keys to the kingdom were now on a computer, rather than on the older, more familiar, card files by Dewey in which I had buried myself for years of academic bliss.

Today I went to the library by myself. The first few times, Dan had gone with me. He helped me use the computer and find my way around. But today I went alone.

It felt really good to reclaim that next piece of me. The digger. The researcher. The thinker. A piece I wasn't sure would come back. But there I was, not only finding more books on desktop publishing than I could ever read, but intuitively finding a book on punch recipes (for the wedding), and a book on the Utah Canyonlands.

There was a deep sense of coming home about the library. Familiar ground. Recognizable terrain. Another subtle piece. Another good tool to put back in my toolbox.

When I reclaimed the library, it felt like I had won a major beachhead victory. It felt as if the Marines were erecting a flag. Knowledge was back within my grasp. The power to assist the thinking process was returned to me, if only in chunks and slivers. I'll take it.

The Dangers of Overachieving

Retraining your brain does not mean making up for lost time. Reframe your thinking to focus on the present. This is not about catching up and recapturing or reclaiming lost opportunity. This is about living your life **now** and about pacing to maintain your quality of lifestyle.

The real trouble sets in if you (who me?) were previously an overachiever because the need to "return to normal" will be more intense. Here is a journal entry from someone I may know, but it certainly is not ME!

JANUARY 16, 1993: ASTROLOGY AND WEAVING, OR HOLDING ONESELF DOUBLY ACCOUNTABLE

Hail the brain-injured overachiever. Who holds herself to a privately contrived standard of performance devoid of human reality or compassion. The double whammy of recovery. A higher standard of performance "under the circumstance" than she would have had when she was "normal" (don't get me started on "normal").

First, there's the over inflated high standard of the average overachiever. Then, seriously overcompensating for the injury on top of the over inflated high standard. Lastly, the double-disappointed and heightened tragedy of having to live below standard and below expectation.

Her self-esteem never had a fighting chance. The view from the inside is that the yardstick grew with the addition of the injury. The normal allowances for impairment are unaccept-able/not valid. The impairment, in fact, escalates and expands performance expectations. The hole digs itself deeper. The overachiever has a higher mark to hit, starting from a lower position.

The trap is set. Recovery time slackens. And this mind-set continues beyond the recovery stage. Even after our heroine has returned to her new self and is performing wonderfully. Her own eyes do not see the result. The belief system about "broken" still runs the show.

I wanted to test my ability to learn. Not in a real school, but just a little class of three-week duration. Something that involved sequencing. I didn't want anyone to know I was going so that, if I failed, there'd be no explaining, no public accountability. So I signed up for an astrology class. Here was a sequencing challenge. Planets, signs, houses, the revolving universe (I can hear those astronomers out there screaming—the universe does not revolve, it expands), the charts, the meanings of the planets depending on what house they are in, retrograde and direct planets, void-of-course moons, planets in opposition/trine/sextile/conjunct, time of day and place you were born: nice, intertwined sequential stuff.

At first I got angry when I didn't understand. Blamed myself for not catching on. Blamed the teacher for being unclear. Then it occurred to me that the other students were struggling, too. And it was just possible that the subject was complicated. What if the topic were complicated? And it all made sense by the third class? What if it wasn't me?

Keep in Mind That You Are OK

Be gentle with yourself. You may have a wacko for an instructor. Just because you don't understand something, does not mean it's about your brain. The subject matter could really be in outer space, or the instruction presented poorly.

More Exercises to Retrain Your Brain

All of the following exercises are meant to offer you different avenues for information retrieval and brain-function enhancement. In each case, assume a comfortable, relaxed position in a quiet and softly lit environment. Begin to relax, closing your eyes, breathing softly. Focus now on your breathing, paying attention as you inhale and exhale. If your mind wanders, just come back to your breathing. Sink deeper into your comfortable position and enjoy the quiet of listening to your breathing. With this approach in mind, choose one of the following exercises and discover how your thinking processes may improve.

The Phone Company Exercise

Is this the party to whom I am speaking? In the days of pioneer telephone operation, switchboards were the norm. Someone in your small town sat at a switchboard and hooked up Aunt Edith and Aunt Bea, and they discussed the town business to their hearts' content.

Well, like it or not, your brain works something like that switchboard. Simplistically, Aunt Edith is your left brain and Aunt Bea is your right brain. The corpus callosum (as seen in the diagram below) connects the two sides of your brain and is the "switchboard" through which the information must travel. When the switchboard is down, yelling across the street is easier than using the phone.

The phone company visualization reconstructs the connections from the two sides of the brain. In your relaxed position as described before, visualize or imagine the two sides of the brain. See or feel the switchboard, much like a screen between the two sides of the brain.

Invite a telephone service guy to each side of the switchboard. Each guy—hard hat, wire, screwdriver, and all—works attentively to establish and repair the connections to the other side. Watch these guys work, and feel or experience that your brain works a little better each time you allow them to work.

Practice this visualization for a few minutes a day. I seemed to think more clearly and feel refreshed after this exercise. Visualization smoothes over a few rough spots.

A→/ B

No Pathway

A⌐/⌐►B

New Pathway

New Pathway with Brain Orienteering

The Office Manager Exercise

Through active imagination, I discovered that, in my head, there was this office manager who was in charge of my collective data. This person resided in a very large office that was crammed with file cabinets, boxes and vaults of papers, and a database file. This person knew where everything was and had the keys to the locked rooms and files, the passwords, and the combinations to the vaults. This person controlled my memory bank.

Learning how to retrieve the information I needed was a matter of getting the office manager to cooperate with my requests. At first, this person was as slow as mud. Depending upon where the answer was filed, a request could take forever and a week to fulfill. With diligence and persistence, however, data retrieval became more and more productive. Here's how it works:

Assume a relaxed position, calming yourself and focusing on your breathing. Picture and imagine in your thoughts a scene of an office, archive, filing room, or control room of some sort. Introduce yourself to the person in charge. Ask her to find a piece of information for you. Make sure it is something that you cannot readily call to mind or that you stumbled with recently.

Watch the process of the manager. Follow her footsteps through the retrieval process. Perhaps you got lost going to work and would like a refresher on the directions. Ask the office manager for a map to the office.

The next time you need a map to the office, go straight to that request, and it will likely be more available to you than it was the previous time. Be as creative as you like. The better the questions, the more productive the answers, and the more exercise you provide your office manager.

You may choose to create a computer format within this framework. Simply include a computer screen in the scenario.

JANUARY 18, 1992

Like a magic wand touched, tapped lightly, and the door simply opened. As if all I had to do was ask.

The Hall Of Answers

Sometimes the simple act of consciously asking a question initiates the path toward the answer.

The Hall of Answers is a great place for data retrieval. Assuming a relaxed position, picture and imagine yourself in a comfortable room, seated in a large and inviting chair. At the end of the room are large double doors. When you are ready, walk toward these doors in your mind, which will open to reveal a long hallway. Along that hallway are many closed doors, along with walls full of little drawers and big drawers.

There are labels on the doors and drawers. Some of the labels are of years, whereas others are of topics. Some drawers hold the names of people, events, or scenes. The drawers are in alphabetic order, and years are in chronologic order. You may ask your questions any way you wish because the answers are cross-referenced.

Ask about what to wear to work. Look under "Power Suit," "Office," "Wardrobe," "Dress for Success," or "Accessories" to offer a few ideas. Can't remember if the blue suit goes with the pink shirt and the orange tie? Consult the Hall of Answers, or at least take off your sunglasses when you get dressed!

When you are ready to conclude your session, come back into the comfortable room and sit back in the large chair. Open your eyes, feeling refreshed and relaxed.

Cross-Crawling Visualization

There will be times when you are too tired or in physical pain and unable to participate in active physical cross-crawling. The good news is that you may visualize your exercise and gain benefit from the work of your thoughts.

Assume a relaxed position, clearing your mind of thought. Follow your breathing. Picture or imagine that you see yourself in your mind's eye. Watch yourself as, in your imagination, you touch your right hand to your left knee, then your left hand to your right knee. Visualize 25 repetitions on each side of your body.

Now, see the cross-crawling pattern as it appears on the front of this book. Visualizing holding the book in your lap, place your right hand on the pattern in your imagination, and trace it with your index finger. Now, reverse the movements so that you trace "backward" of your first pattern. Now repeat those movements, visualizing using your left hand.

Make sure that, in your visualization, your hand and arm cross past the midline of the body. Past your nose-to-bellybutton line, as it were. (You remember Aunt Edith and Aunt Bea and the switchboard? The same rules apply here. Crossing the midline equals hooking up the switchboard.

Very good thing to do.) Once you are familiar with this exercise, let your imagination create as many different tracing patterns as you like.

When you are finished, focus again on your breathing, open your eyes, and feel refreshed and renewed.

Progressive Muscle Relaxation

There are numerous progressive relaxation tapes on the market. Your psychotherapist, hypnotherapist, contemporary bookstore, librarian, massage therapist, or an alternative lifestyle catalog will be able to direct you to effective ones.

Progressive relaxation basically means that the body is incrementally relaxed through visualization and muscle awareness. Traditionally, the toes are relaxed first, then the legs and arms, progressing through the body to the head, scalp, and eyelids. It all feels really good and may serve to relax you. It is definitely sound therapy for brain-injury recovery. It is a classic external trigger to body awareness and peace.

I'm OK Today Exercise

Assume a comfortable and relaxed position. Focus on your breathing and begin to feel warm. Allow these thoughts to come into your being, giving them room to grow inside: My body attracts gentle healing. I am OK just the way I am. My energy is used wisely by my body to heal my brain. I am willing to do what I need to do to support my healing process. I am OK today. Everything I do supports and contributes to my well-being. I take naps and eat wisely to support my healing process. Who I am today is enough. What I accomplish today is enough. The energy I have today is enough. My abundant energy is spent wisely on my healing process. I attract help and support. I am OK today.

Continue breathing, relaxing and hearing these words: I support my healing process by living one day at a time. I ask for support and receive support easily. I am OK today. I let go of my old beliefs about life. I embrace my new life. I embrace the new me. I am OK today. I love myself as I heal my body. I attract loving support. I am lovable just as I am today. I am OK today.

It is helpful if you use one affirmation at a time or if a friend reads these affirmations to you while you relax. When you are ready to conclude this exercise, focus on your breathing and allow your eyes to open. You feel refreshed and peaceful.

Gadgets and Games

New technologies emerge daily that support recovery of cognitive function. Along with the relaxation tapes and DVDs for visualization, yoga, tai chi, chi gong, and meditation sessions, you may also find video games like Journey to Wild Divine, which are calming and teach relaxation with biofeedback-like sensors on your fingers.

When choosing computer-based technologies, refrain from loud, noisy, violent, flashing, or visually taxing applications. Limit your use to 10 minutes a day, and build your play time and stamina slowly. Consider turning off the sound or wearing ear plugs while you play to soften the audio effect on your ears.

Choose your technology applications carefully and work with them slowly to build your abilities.

Summary

Visualization and cross-crawling are very powerful tools of repair, retrieval, and remembering. They can be used daily to build and strengthen the pathways in your brain. Stimulate your brain. Provide external triggers. Watch classic movies, funny cartoons, the Three Stooges, game shows, or Mr. Science for familiar remembering.

You have not forgotten anything. It is all in there. It may be in a vault, and the key may be lost, but it is in there. You just need a better map, a road crew, a technician, a manager, a filing system, or a trip to the video store to unlock the way.

22

Remembering
What You Know

There are moments when you want to retrieve a morsel of information and you know you know it, but it won't come forward. You cannot get to it. "I hear you knocking, but you can't come in."

Remembering what you know is a process of reminding, accessing, and retrieving your knowledge. Repeating and modeling from external stimuli is very helpful. (See the chapter "Retrain Your Brain.")

External Modeling

When you remind yourself of what you know by external example to jog your memory, you are practicing external modeling. The external stimulus is the item or action so used.

Remembering Who You Are

I, for instance, am a mountain climber. I hike, camp, ski, Orienteer, climb, and fill my heart with joy in the mountains. Sitting on the couch is not for me. This journal entry is my first hankering to return to my life.

JULY 2, 1991

Enough of this recovery already. The red meat, the couch, the heat, the tired, the walks. I want a mountain to sink my teeth into.

Another week and a half on the couch, then exercise. And a taste of altitude, if you please.

Champagne for the nostrils. Breathe it in, long, tingling, and thin. Crisp, cool, and under-oxygenated. Makes you breathe deeper to get what you need. So crisp, so light, so ... wonderful.

The high air. I smell it with my soul. It feeds me, nourishes me, heals me in a way that encircles my being and energizes me, molecule by grateful molecule. Has cabin fever ever been so poetic? Bordering on lustful? Downright lusting for tree line?

The flowers are blooming without me to smell them. I gotta go up. Take me.

Television

Your television set can be a powerful tool in your recovery. It can bring the world to you, quiz you, entertain you, provide you with a safe place to be, and offer you companionship. In your healthy state, that reflects a dismal view of life. But now, it can be your friend and your path back to what you know. Remember to screen for TV overload and only watch when your energy level is capable of it.

JANUARY 28, 1993: MY TV

The TV helped. Old movies to remind me where I come from. Jeopardy and Wheel of Fortune to help me remember what I know. Bullwinkle and Rocky to help me laugh. CNN for world view. The Food Channel and HGTV. Oprah to make me think. Dave and Jay for company in the evenings. No soap operas, just not my style. Meet the Press occasionally. And the Comedy Channel.

And I'd turn it off a lot, too. Short attention span being what it is. And take naps.

My living room window was a marvelous TV, too. I watched spring turn into summer, saw the flowers bloom, the maple leaf, the catalpa spread her orchid-like flowers across the sky of the yard and send her intoxicating fragrance inside to comfort me.

One afternoon, after the thunder and showers had subsided, and the air cleared, a mother skunk and her brood took a tour through the neighborhood, down the sidewalk in front of me, these busy balls of fluff on a mission, exploring the sniffs, keeping up with mom, showing off her pride and joy.

I knew something was up when all the cats, squirrels, and dogs were suddenly absent and silent. This private parade, held just for me. It was a precious moment.

Bring It Back Alive

Refresh and tune up your brain with little bits of information any time you can. There is abundant stored information captive inside your brain, and an external trigger may spark it forward into the useful memory realm. Always worth a try.

Summary

Remembering what you know is dynamic in restoring your brain power and supporting the healing process. Discover the triggers your brain craves.

23

Humor

The brain focuses primary attention on the processes that are easiest to restore. Then the repair work appears to move to the more complicated and less vital functions. Humor, for instance, is a central part of my life. But humor is a very complicated mental process not vital to survival.

Laughter communicates powerfully. That's why it is so troublesome when you don't get a joke, or you laugh late.

This chapter reminds us of the power and complexity of humor. When the jokes return, you know real progress is being made. (Yes, record that one in the journal!)

Humor

For openers, humor requires sequencing. Humor also requires metaphor, symbolism, reference, play on words, and cultural or social nuance. Most importantly, humor requires timing. When your brain is healing, there is no time for any of this silliness. Humor is out.

In short, humor requires focused and coordinated energy. When your energy pie is running a quart low, you will not be able to process humor. It is too exhausting.

So there you are at a party, listening to people tell stories, jokes, and puns. Suddenly everyone bursts into belly laughter. You are clueless. Your eyes are glazed over as your brain struggles to process and make sense of the data. You are linear. There is no hope.

Half an hour later, when your brain has finally worked this little joke through your head (while dealing with the noise, lights, swimming faces, and sensory overload of the party), you laugh.

When Humor Returns

Because of its complicated nature, the return of your sense of humor is a definitive sign of progress and success.

JUNE 28, 1991

The jokes are beginning to sink in now. I'm now more aware of the missing puzzle pieces. I know when I'm "not following" now. Still can't quite keep up, but I remember the quickness now that once was present.

My sense of former self is coming into focus now. So the patchy self-exam begins. What was good from the old life? What to keep, what to toss. What to adjust, what to tuck in a bit.

If I had a second shot at life, what would I do ... now? What? And when? And how?

The compulsion, not to blame or judge, but to change, alter, improve, polish, or wish a bigger wish. Really go for it (whatever it is), really reach, really grasp, really ... what? Am I missing something here?

What? What is the haunting thought? What is the urge, the need; what is the unasked question? The inertia for a "more" than there was before. And what about the peace I felt when I agreed to die? It was fine with me. Quiet, peaceful, a good day to die. And yet, here I am. Shall the return be as arbitrary as the fall? Shall I simply come back, innocently, graciously, as peacefully as I would have gone?

Is peace the final gift? The final state? Is peace my gift? Can it be that easy? That simple? To be at peace. On the couch, eating red meat, watching my vacations go by, watching the hikers, bikers, campers, and river rafts float by, and be at peace with that. To watch my body take small, decisive, and positive healing steps every day. To unfold layer by layer, level by level, brain cell by brain cell, day by sunny day, and to be at peace with it.

To trust. Let go. Rely upon. Receive. To place myself in God's hands and accept the love in all the forms it has taken these five weeks. I don't know. And yet ... my short-term memory is working just enough to drive me crazy. I may not have disability insurance, but I have peace of mind. Peace of heart. Peace of spirit.

How did all this succeed in filling my bucket? In a few more weeks, when my mind is working better, I'll probably be able to say something profound.

Laughter

I consider laughter a cornerstone of personal happiness. To view the world with a grain of salt is a powerful position. Laughing your way back to good humor is a tried and true therapy technique. Viewing classic comedy will remind you of the style of humor present in our culture. External modeling of comedy provides hours of fun and therapy at the same time.

The video and DVD store overflows with comedy. Everything from The Three Stooges to Lily Tomlin and Steve Martin will offer you a window back into what you enjoy.

And with video, remember, if you don't get the joke, just rewind the tape and play it again. Not to mention the "outtakes" on DVDs. Wonderful. What could be more convenient?

Allow yourself to laugh. Work toward laughing at yourself. Nothing provides grace, personal acceptance, and rebuilt self-esteem faster than personal perspective.

Practice Telling a Joke

Find a joke book in the library or have someone tell you a joke. Write it down and practice it. Tell the joke to a friend and see how it goes. If it goes well, she will laugh. If you botch it, laugh at yourself!

The Day Humor Came Back

More on the continuing saga of my trip to the writer's workshop in Utah.

NOVEMBER 9, 1992: TUNA SALAD

Today I was labeled the class cut-up. It's been a very long time since last I engaged in comedy. It, too, was a piece of me misplaced by the accident.

Oh, I've seen smidgens of it poking its rubber nose and mustache over the fence from time to time, a redundant pun here, a noise or slide down the banister there. But only pieces of a rich quiet that once kept me warmly cozy and amused.

For a long while, I have stood now just to one side of the proscenium, missing the timing, seeing the humor amble too late through the lines in the twinkle of my eye. I've chuckled a lot to myself this last year and a half, the only one laughing at my jokes, torturous seconds and sometimes minutes post facto. At least I was laughing, but laughing alone. Even with the laughing came the tragedy within, the missed moment and the memory of my former witty and quite often knee-slapping, gut-painful, teary-eyed regale (ah, another marginal and unintentional pun. My relief is growing).

How does the old line go? "Of all the things I've lost, I miss my mind the most" or as former V.P. Dan Quayle so aptly put it to the NAACP, "A mind is a terrible thing to lose."

Wanting to smile, to share that smile with others, had lost the place inside me it used to come from. I was somber. But I wanted/needed to smile, so the painted-on smile and the darker lipstick helped, but my jaws and cheeks ached by the end of the day. Especially after work. People were coming to me for help. I was the well, happy, and adjusted wise woman. I smiled. It hurt. But I made myself do it. So hoping that the external behavior pattern would trigger my lost friend to wake up and come back out to play again.

Other memories, other pieces, other lost chunks of the puzzle had been triggered and come back; why were the jokes taking so long?

Yes, I can hear you all screaming the answer: because humor isn't funny. It's a very subtle and discerning process requiring timing, sequencing, cognitive reasoning, and speed mixed with intellectual acuity and a level of omniscient perspective that takes in the bigger picture and the connecting nuance, all in a split moment of elegant timing. Yes, it's more complicated than remembering how to can apricots. Or adding columns of figures.

What do I have to do to get it back? I miss the laughing that only a belly can convey.

Pack Creek Ranch served lunch and was very gracious to label their offerings; on the back of a business card, it read "Tuna Salad." Susan Tweit, desert naturalist and seminar leader extra ordinaire, seized this card with tape attached and was of a mind to tape it to my back, but somehow I turned about, intercepted it, and placed it on my shirt pocket where my name tag should have been.

Tuna Salad. A solid name. I wore it a while, deciding that this writers' conference was entirely too earnest, too intense, not light enough, not—well, damn it—funny enough. So I slipped the new name tag in my old one and began wearing *it* in earnest.

Somehow it all triggered and I became Tuna Salad. But not just any tuna salad. The Rev. Dr. Tuna Salad to you. The laughing was delicious. I was delighted, embarrassed, and tearfully joyful to have created the noise. It felt good to bring glee to a room again. The funny girl was back. I was accused of being the class cut-up. It was music to my ears.

Summary

Humor is good. Real progress accompanies a good punch line. Journal the day. Write down the joke. Write down how good it felt to laugh. You have arrived at a cognitively complex moment. Savor it.

24

Power Nap

When your body tells you to rest, you had best listen. The power center of your brain will arm wrestle you and win. If you persist, unfocused vision, slurred speech, stumbled step, and heavy eyelids are in your future. No intellectual argument will overcome the command. Surrender.

This chapter discusses the absolute necessity for profound, frequent, and nonnegotiable napping. The amount of rest needed to heal the brain is many times more necessary than for other injuries. Your brain will get you to rest, one way or the other. Cooperation is extremely important. Learn the advantages of the power nap.

Power Nap

I call this the power nap for two reasons. One, because taking a nap gives you the necessary energy to continue with your day. Two, because overachievers need to think they are doing something powerful, even when horizontal. The power nap may be a true sleeping event or it may simply be a private, peaceful and prone eyes closed in a quiet place kind of experience. Key characteristics: quiet, eyes closed, lying down.

Surrender Dorothy!

Surrender to the power of your brain to *make* you rest. There will be clues. Pay attention. You need a nap when

○   Your vision blurs more than usual

○   Your speech slurs more than usual

○   Your attention span takes a dive

○   Your motor skills decrease (you stumble, feel weak, drop things)

○   Your eyes have increased sensitivity to light

○   You have a headache

○   The world appears to be in slow motion

○   Your emotions are shut down

○   Your emotions blow up

○   Your body suddenly feels chilled

○   Your brain shuts down

As an overachiever, I struggled with the nap thing. Naps used to be what you did after lunch in the summer so you wouldn't get cramps at the pool and drown. So much for transient wisdom.

MARCH 23, 1993

I struggled before I surrendered.

My eyes still don't work all the time. They just quit focusing. So rest, I tell myself.

Tell a race horse to take a nap. High performance is an interesting habit to break. When peak performance is your normal state of being and you lose a slice of it, that hunk of you that you miss isn't obvious or even apparent to those around you. (Now you tell me.)

And rest the only cure. Time the only medicine. Patience the long-term verdict. And me with so much to do, so many directions to turn, so much to share and explore. Knowing full well that rest is my prison and my friend.

How to Take a Power Nap

A beneficial power nap has to last as long as it needs to. Your brain has taken you down for the count. Cooperation is vital. The nap may last 15 minutes or two hours.

Rest in as horizontal a position as possible. Putting your head on your desk will not suffice. I am talking bed, sofa, recliner with blanket, pillow, and loosened clothes. Teddy bear is optional. Darkened room, telephone and pager off, quiet environment. Do not disturb.

Sleep is possible but not necessary. Quiet rest also qualifies. Eyes closed at all times. Shoes off, glasses off. A real nap. A total time out.

Power Nap Exercise

Find a dark, comfortable place with a couch, bed, or reclining chair for resting. Keep a blanket or afghan nearby. Loosen tight clothing, unbuckle belts, remove shoes and glasses, find your pillow, and assume a restful and relaxing position. Turn off the lights, phone, answering machine, and beeper. Close your eyes and begin to relax your feet. Allow the muscles of your feet and legs to grow heavy. Let the feeling of heaviness travel up your legs to your pelvis. As the heaviness travels, your body feels warm and comfortable. Allow the muscles of your back to relax, feeling the bed press against them. Breathe deeply and release the chest muscles. Exhale with relief, sinking deeper into the mattress.

Feel your fingers becoming warm and heavy, and let that relaxing, heavy feeling travel up your arms to your shoulders. Let your neck relax, then your head, scalp, and jaw. Continue breathing deeply as the muscles of your face, lips, and eyes also become heavy and warm. With your next breath, allow a wave of relaxation to move from your head to your toes, allowing you to sink deeper into the bed. Allow this wave of relaxation to repeat itself several times, until you are completely relaxed and willing to rest deeply. Drift gently to restful sleep. Your Power Nap has begun.

Observe your own personal needs. It is not unreasonable to nap several times a day in the early months of recovery. Two good naps a day after a year or two is still within normal range of need. You may be able to taper off to occasional naps after that, depending upon your individual requirements. Once napping interferes with successful nighttime sleep, re-evaluate.

Sleep

Are you sleeping? Getting 7 to 8 hours of uninterrupted, peaceful, and restorative sleep? Do you awaken refreshed? Remember to report poor, unfulfilling, or uneven sleep patterns to your doctor.

Occasionally, mild brain injury contributes to sleep disruption or disturbed sleep patterns. Perhaps your brain struggles to "turn off'" so you can sleep or you wake up in the middle of the night and your brain kicks in. These frustrations can be a part of brain injury that deals with sleep disturbance or sleep disorders. A sleep study may be helpful.

Getting good sleep that matches with the natural rhythm of your body is very important. Consider the various approaches to obtaining restful sleep suggested by your doctors.

Summary

Listen to your brain. The more proficient you become at identifying and honoring the clues of your impending nap, the more powerfully useful the nap is, and the less time you waste struggling against the inevitable. Surrender. Nap.

Any time can be nap time.

25

A Good Brain Day

There is a light at the end of the tunnel, and I call it "A Good Brain Day." That's a day that progressed smoothly, with no appreciable exhaustion at the end. That's a day to remember. Also a day not to take for granted. Journal it.

Have a Good Brain Day!

A day will come when the clouds will lift and regular events will follow one another. On that day, you will perceive yourself in a state of wellness. Everything will go your way. There will be no stumbling, no slurred words, no panic, no lost time or lost directions. The day you have been waiting for will slip into your life unannounced.

Be sure to record it. Write down all the great things that happened. List the smooth sense of gliding through your day. Note your clear thinking. Note the happy smile on your face.

The following day will predictably be a relapse day. Your journal will be most valuable in reminding you that a good brain day is not only possible, but likely to return. Your future now begins to contain good brain days. If you can have one, you will have more.

Soon you will link good days together and have two or three in a row before your brain decides to refuel. In time, an entire week will contain smooth and normal life.

TRUCKERS DON'T BE FOOLED. YOU STILL HAVE MILES TO GO

This is one of my favorite signs on Interstate 70 just west of Denver. It warns the uninitiated 18-wheeler that there is more work to be done. The truckers aren't off the mountain yet. And neither are you.

A good brain day soon becomes a good brain week, then a good brain month.

WARNING: Avoid complacency. You may forget your vulnerability and return to your overachiever lifestyle. Expect a relapse, most likely of the bushwhacking variety. Seemingly from nowhere, various refueling symptoms may sweep down upon you. This happens. It feels familiar. It will pass.

Out there on the edge of the Energy Pie, not all of the borders are completely defined. Time for a nap. Time to remember that this setback is still a part of the healing process. Gear down. Stay in the slow lane. Pay attention to the terrain. You are not off the mountain yet.

Success Is at Hand

Once you start to have good brain weeks and months, the overall process of healing is definitely on the upswing. The good times begin to outweigh the challenging times. The light at the end of the tunnel really is sunshine. Stay mindful that you remain vulnerable. Keep a modest vigilance on your energy.

The Fuzzy Brain Day

Halfway between a Good Brain Day and a difficult brain day is the Fuzzy Brain Day. It is like being in limbo: not bad, not great, just hazy, fuzzy, and dim. On those days, clear thinking is tedious. Chores like laundry, loading the dishwasher, or light cleaning can be accomplished, but little else.

Fuzzy days are the days I go for a walk, tidy up a room, iron shirts, and clean the kitchen. I might as well. These chores are the most productive use of my time and energy for a fuzzy day. I found that I felt more competent and productive once I accepted fuzzy days and adapted certain tasks to those times.

Fuzzy days are just another state of being with regard to brain injury. I just do what I can under daily circumstances. Fuzzy Days are a good sign of incremental recovery.

Summary

A Good Brain Day is a wonderful thing. Soak it up. Remember it. Record it.

26

Journaling

Writing about your healing journey on a daily basis is extremely helpful for your brain. Recording your thoughts, your progress, your feelings and disappointments, your anger, and your successes is very important. You have been reading my journal entries throughout this book. I wrote in my journal frequently, especially when I had something significant or useful to record about my recovery.

Keeping a journal using paper and pen will remind you that you can write. It keeps you alert to your retained talents. Journaling triggers your memory about what you know. It performs a "cross-crawl" function for the brain and calls you to external daily contact with cognitive thought.

This chapter shows you how to journal your way back to yourself. Your journal gives you a safe place to be every day with the only person who really understands: you!

Journal Your Brain Back

This is about writing. Not typing or computer voice recognition. Writing with pen or pencil on paper makes you cross the midline of your body, and it reinforces your spelling and learning. Sit with the paper before you, turned at a comfortable angle to your body. Write by hand. To do this you must focus, spell, think, and express. Notice that you are writing!

Journaling Position for Cross-Crawling Benefit

Hold your journal on your lap or position it on a table or writing surface in such a way that, in order to write, your pen in hand crosses past your belly button (as seen in the diagram on the facing page).

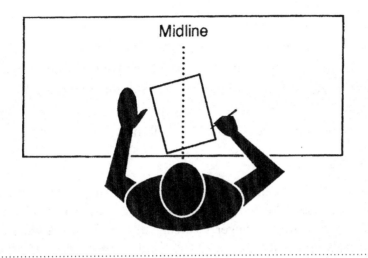

Cross-Crawl Diagram with Midline

JANUARY 28, 1993

Crying a lot? Can't see any changes, REAL changes? Forgot all those words you paid good money to learn? Buy a green steno pad, like the one I wrote this book on, and start journaling. Or writing. Or taking notes. It will help you track your progress.

This is not busy work. This is vital. Hold the pad across your lap so you get some cross-meridian benefit. Write down your feelings. All the unattractive stuff about being broken, at sea, unconnected, unsexy, lost, unheard. About wondering if not being here would have been easier. About losing your partner because you're not the person she or he married. About losing yourself, and not knowing who you are now. About "why me?" About sitting and staring. About the world being a different place. And choices and priorities looking different.

Or write a letter and let someone know what it's like. How you feel. The good, the bad, the ugly. I remember the day I could add again. And when my nipples woke up. And when I solved a complex therapeutic puzzle. And when I remembered how to put on eye shadow.

But I remember these events in part because I wrote them down and dated them. Recorded events, and your improved use of language, reinforce your recovery. Misspell words. Use bad grammar. Turn nouns into verbs. Dangle those participles. Whatever. Just communicate. Tell jokes. Draw. Doodle. Speak your truth. What you have to say is not debatable or negotiable. Write. Practice signing your name. Write a one-line affirmation (like: "I'm OK, just the way I am" and "I am enough"). Do it.

Write down what happens to you every day. It may be a brief line, a paragraph, or a splash of run-on sentences. Be sure to record daily triumphs, agonies, and subtle improvements. Talk about your general mood and any nuances you may be feeling. If you are a professional journal writer or diary keeper and think this journaling exercise just reminds you of a skill you have lost, reframe the experience. Feel free to call this effort "recording."

MAY 12, 1992

> Journaling has been therapy. Writing down my feelings. Noticing that I spell better than before. That sentences are easier. That I can write for longer stretches of time. That the ideas and concepts flow onto the page. That I can read it later and follow along. I feel sad. For the loss. Glad. For the recovering. Scared. For what might not return. Lost. To memories that lacked priority. Hopeful that enough will trigger my memory that those precious, noncritical pieces will come back. Nuances of my son's early life. Jokes with great punch lines.
>
> No more stuttering. No more slurred or compact new words. No more pain. Just thought. My thought. Smooth, energetic, creative, dynamic thought, the real me. The old real me. Who am I? Who was I?

Journaling helps you notice and remember how far you have come and that improvements, however subtle, continue to take place. Journaling also gives you a place to express all the thoughts and events that happen to you in contrast to your surroundings, and in contrast to the past.

Journaling gives you a place to be OK, a safe place to reside emotionally. Writing down your day lets you be OK just as you are today. It provides a first place to discover the new you, with any luck at all. Your journal is a great place to write down humorous inhibition stories, which will probably be funny six months from now. Especially write down the "oh my God" stories.

MAY 23, 1992

> My mind seems paralyzed. Life in limbo. The days fly by and I stand still. Quietly.
>
> It's been a year, today, since I fell. I'm here, alive. Recovering financially. Recovering mentally. Healing in bits and pieces still. The flashbacks of the accident float in and remind me that I'm still in therapy—it's not over.

I can't seem to get back to physical activity. The TV is on a lot lately. Before I never watched. Now, I look to it to shift my thinking and take care of me.

My body has reshaped but holds 25 pounds of weight that I seem to be hanging on to. I'm still moved to tears easily. Especially this week as all the reminders of the accident loom large.

Journal, because your mind is a sieve and you will appreciate these thoughts later.

Buy Sticky Notes and a Franklin Day Planner

Luckily there are sticky notes. Buy a stack of them and use them all you want. Everyone else does. No one will read yours.

Once you have mastered the sticky notes, you may wish to consider a Franklin Day Planner. I was a very organized person before I began to use this tool. Now I am even more efficient and effective. I can keep track of my life. Everything I need to know is in one place. (See "Resources.")

The Day I Could Add in my Head Again

It may not seem like very much, but, to me, adding figures in my head is an important skill. Priding myself as a card-carrying Black Belt Shopper, knowing what it all costs is vital to knowing whether I can afford my prizes.

The brain injury took that skill away. Two plus two was written down and performed on paper. A year and a half after the accident, I was in Breckenridge, Colorado, attending an International Avalanche meeting. Helping out at the registration and T-shirt counter, I was selling shirts, commemorative mugs, and lapel pins. It suddenly occurred to me that I was adding purchases in my head.

I was thrilled. Surrounded by snow physicists from all over the world, I had no one to share my triumph. "I can add again! I can add again!" seemed inappropriate and out of context. Sharing it with my journal gave me a place to go and to record my modest victory. I recaptured another skill. Record. Remember where I have been, and where I have yet to travel.

OCTOBER 4, 1992

Today I was able to add single columns of numbers without having to struggle or write it down and check it. The doubt seemed to have lifted. I just went ahead and added two T-shirts and a mug together and came up with the answer. It felt good. Notation of another returned skill. A sigh of relief and on to the next sale! A small improvement; another piece of the puzzle; a parcel of myself returned—long gone, found, and back in place. It seems a small enough issue. Small pieces are all that seem left now: tiny parts, slivers of me, prickles on my skin like walking through thistles and trying to wash off the stings. Phantom stings, illusive yet painful enough. I know they're still there. Little stings, fading but not slowly enough. Fading, stinging, itching, scratching. Emotional Calamine, self-esteem lotion to soothe the wait."

Journaling Is Inspirational

Your journal is a clear picture of your trek toward recovery and the new revealing YOU. When I first began to journal this recovery, it was a pure expression of my pain, my agony, my anger, my frustration, my rage, and my flopping about on the beach. I needed someone to talk to.

My journal did not start out to be this book. It was my way to reach inside and pull out my *self* so that I could look at her and begin to figure out the new *her*! This woman was experiencing and expressing thoughts and emotions that the old me did not easily recognize as being ME. I wanted to know what was going on. I wanted some understanding, if not control.

Journaling was my way to make sense of my predicament.

AUGUST 4, 1992

There have been many dry years, years without really writing, years of notes and paragraphs dated and held for later. Stacked on the desk. Waiting.

Waiting, but for what? Or Whom? Or When? I wasn't sure but it hadn't arrived yet, I was sure enough of that. It felt mostly like there were three books swimming about in my head like synchronized lilies awaiting their music. Three, each of a different color, wondering how this dance would play itself out. The degree of difficulty seeming high. The squinting judges just beyond the mist.

Waiting.

I'm a cook. A holy woman. A philosopher and healer. A skier and a lover. Metaphysician and black belt shopper.

Waiting. Writing while I wait. Watching, listening and growing while I wait.

The Lord blesses those who wait. Being of the "worketh like helleth while I waiteth" school of patience, I figured I'd be prepared when the spontaneity showed up.

Then a woman died. A woman I'd never heard of. But plenty of people knew of her and she was eulogized by those I respect. So I began to seek her books and found what I had been waiting for: a kindred spirit, a mentor of sorts.

Someone, in M.F.K. Fisher, who wrote the way I've been wanting to write but had no successful model. A brief scanning of "How to Cook a Wolfe" and my final puzzle pieces fell into place. Her honest, crisp style merged with me as if I had known her for years. In her passing, she has gifted me with a glimpse of myself. I am grateful and relieved. I can proceed now. Perhaps what I have to say and the manner in which it is delivered shall honor her as it enriches you. I am enriched by the doing.

The overall point is a sense of artistic companionship. I am no longer alone. Until my discovery, isolation continued to take a large bite out of my resolve to write.

Knowing that intuition and style are my pure modes of expression, then revealing that stance , seemed worlds apart, before Mary Frances, my new imaginary friend, appeared.

Now I know how Calvin feels, comforted by Hobbes as he reveals his innermost schemings to the universe and one friendly ear. Companionship is a precious commodity. Not for sale at any price. And once found, not negotiable.

Should I write every day whether or not I'm so inspired? Well, no, generally. All those writing books insist on daily practice, but is it really for the discipline of it? I tend to write when I think I have something to say. Entirely likely that I'm no judge of that! Oh well. I write when I feel so moved. The tablet is never far, however. By the bed, at the desk, in the suitcase while on the move.

Summary

Write it down, no matter how big, little, weird, funny, seemingly inconsequential, or discounted it may seem at the time. One line could reward you with a solved puzzle piece six months from now! Write it down. Date it.

Keep your tablet close. I like the green stenographers' tablets best. And a pen will clip nicely into the wire binding, always handy.

Here's a simplified method for convenient journaling.

Get help to build your own notebook with premade sheets of paper prompting you to respond on several items. Then, you just fill them out. It will seem more like a questionnaire than a journal. Possible line items to consider: date, medical appointments, medical news of progress, mental state, physical state, emotional state, spiritual state, I feel......, I want......, I tried this......, I succeeded......., today for the first time in a long time, I..........., this is better. Please add others that are appropriate for you.

Thoughts, people who brightened my day. My favorite color, smell, taste, or scene of the day. Most interesting texture. Favorite food of the day. This is fun!

Part V

THE PHYSICAL BODY

"Basically, your eyes suck energy like a toaster."
G. Denton

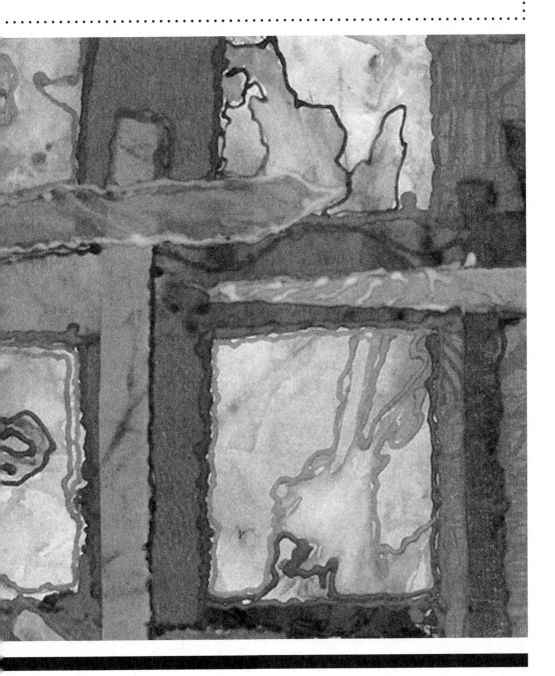

27

Physical Issues

Certain physical issues may accompany mild brain injury, whether or not you sustained bodily injury in your accident. You may be experiencing problems with balance, dizziness, or "vestibular" problems. Nausea, neck pain, headaches, blurred vision, jaw clenching or teeth grinding in your sleep, scalp aches, neck and shoulder pain, carpal tunnel trigger to the forearms, upper back pain, uneven swallowing, choking on saliva while inhaling, or choking on small bits of food may occur. Your glasses prescription, as well as your sleeping cycles, hormonal cycles, and digestive processes, may change.

This chapter considers possible body changes that you may experience temporarily.

Desensitizing to Your Systems Being Overwhelmed

When brain injury occurs, not only the noticeable, but also the subtle systems of the body become overwhelmed. The Western medical model tries to isolate and treat the head. The holistic medical model observes that when one part of the body is affected, all parts are affected. Brain injury is a perfect example of the whole body being affected by an injury to "just one place."

When the brain is injured, the entire body feels like it is on "red alert." It seems as if "everything" is sensitive. In many cases, this is true. For some people, only certain systems are affected. Each individual response is different. Some overwhelmed systems feed into the overload of another system, and the complex becomes magnified. If it sounds like a big mess, it is. And it isn't much fun either. This chapter will list a number of symptomatic problems that you may or may not experience, or that you may experience to a greater or lesser degree than others.

This chapter will help to let you know that you are not crazy and that you are not making up physical symptoms. And it will let you know that your pain or sensitivity is not "in your head" but may very well be a result of your brain injury. The good news is that these systems will desensitize over time and that they tend to regulate themselves again. Other chapters in the book will show you how to enhance the desensitization process. Consult the index for more help by using the headings in this chapter as your guide.

Vestibular Abilities

Balance, dizziness, and nausea are examples of vestibular ability. Can you walk straight, stand up quickly, and maintain balance? Can you close your eyes and touch your nose with your outstretched hand? Do you often feel slightly nauseous? Sources for these experiences may be the inner ear or the cervical stability of the neck. Consider soft tissue therapies, osteopathy, craniosacral technique, and chiropractic care to reduce symptoms.

Dizziness can be constant, or it may come and go. Until it wears off, refrain from driving a vehicle or operating kitchen machines. Moving slowly can help. Consider wearing sunglasses and a brimmed hat all the time.

Vision

Have your eyes become overly sensitive to light? Is your vision blurred? Are there black spots or areas of your scope of sight that are fuzzy or gone? Can you see peripherally? When you can see, has your ability to focus been altered? Do you feel like your glasses' prescription needs to be changed? Have you resorted to wearing sunglasses all day, even in the house?

This all sounds in line with brain-injury symptoms. Wearing sunglasses is a great idea because your eyes may be "photophobic," or sensitive to light. If you wear prescription glasses or contacts, they may not be working as well as they used to.

It is important to see a neurologist and an eye specialist (preferably a holistic or behavioral ophthalmologist) during this time because your eyes may progressively change their ability several times during your recovery.

A trick that helps me when I really need to use my eyes for short, important functions, like threading a needle, is to take a few deep breaths to flush my system with oxygen. My eyes improve their acuity temporarily with this procedure, especially if I don't abuse the privilege.

Hormones

The true guardians of body function, the cycles regulated by hormones, include sleep, wakeful time, sex, sexual cycles, body-cycle regularity, digestion, elimination, menstrual cycle, brain cycles, body rhythms, and secretions of all sorts. Hormones are the workhorses of the body and the choreographers of daily rhythms.

You may not sleep well at night. You may not be able to digest food well or routinely eliminate bodily waste products. Your menstrual cycle may go off schedule and take years to return to its routine.

Germ-wise, your immune system may be less able to fight off invaders, especially the low-grade variety. Yeast infections, enzyme imbalances, dandruff, bowel flora, colds, coughs, and other hangers-on may take months to eradicate. This, by itself, can be exhausting. Guarding the immune system is vital. Consult a naturopathic or homeopathic physician.

Sex

You may experience a disinterest in sex or a temporary inability to function sexually. Sexual activity is a complicated bodily activity, so having sex, like telling jokes (see the chapter "Humor") takes systems cooperation to be successful. Further, since it is not a vital function of the body, compared to breathing, for instance, the brain can put sex aside in favor of activities linked with immediate survival and recovery.

Although this may not be great news, at least the future will be better once the brain has extra energy to devote to more complicated tasks. Sex, like humor, will return to your life.

At first, you may notice that your sexual function is not quite as you remembered it. The brain may need external modeling. Practice is good. (See the chapter "Sexual Response.") Your overall energy or stamina may alter your experience, too. Enjoy the intimacy and contact.

TMJ

The temporomandibular joints, or the joints that hold the jaw to the skull, can endure serious stress, strain, and injury in conjunction with brain injury. You may begin or increase the habit of clenching your teeth at night, simply from the stress of your brain injury. This can not only injure your teeth, but also significantly increase tenderness in your jaw joint. You may wish to consult a dentist for a therapeutic oral splint. It will decrease injury to the teeth and may ease tenderness in your jaw joint. I highly recommend a lower-jaw splint rather than the more common upper splint. The lower-jaw splint is less stressful to the sutures of the skull and gentler to the jaw joint. It does require more dental skill to make. Don't let the dentist pooh-pooh your request. Consult a massage therapist, craniosacral practitioner, osteopath, or chiropractor for therapies to reduce pain.

Headaches and Face Pain

Pain generally associated with headaches may occur, and it may occur in many ways. This may be caused by TMJ, a general injury reaction from your accident, or a general response to stress in your body. Facial pain likewise can occur from these sources. You may also experience "eye aches," scalp aches, and even pain while thinking.

Warm towels to the face can help, as can biofeedback techniques and relaxation visualization. Over-the-counter medications may or may not assist, depending upon your metabolism. Consider craniosacral therapy, soft tissue therapy, acupuncture, and chiropractic.

Snoring

You may add new behaviors to your life as well. Snoring, for instance, may enter your life. Oh, well. This too may pass.

DECEMBER 16, 1991: THERE IS SOMETHING IN MY THROAT.

> Snoring is another matter entirely, or so it seemed. Over the years of tension, other less obvious supportive body parts joined in the

twilight fun. Tensing, holding, transferring pain to and from the jaw, through the neck, to the chest and upper back. At least, this is the osteopath's theory. The jaw let go, but the throat (unaware of the release order from above) continues to stand guard.

So, deep in sleep, the jaw (usually clenched tight) now opens easily and gently. The cool bedroom air then jostles its way down the throat, gurgling and harmonizing on its way, chiming in to arouse the gentle sleeper at my side.

Not a legal snore, per se. A tense throat, sore next morning from overwork. Not a nasal or sinus echo. Just my throat, needing the same respite from old ways long since guarded against by the mandible. At least he says it's a cute snore.

A theory worth a try. Another layer peeled away. Uncovering what lies beneath, always a surprise. Peel the next one. Snore on!

Swallowing

Your swallowing reflex may alter, and the chance of choking or inhaling saliva may increase. You may notice that you choke on food more frequently, involuntarily regurgitate small amounts of food, or inhale instead of swallow food or drink. Swallowing requires a coordination activity, like humor or sex.

Be alert and focus on your food while eating and drinking. Distraction such as socializing can cause overload and you may choke on food, drink, or saliva.

It is not uncommon to experience regurgitation, and a hiatal hernia may be the source. This could be caused from the force of an accident. With indigestion as an issue, it is important to keep an eye on the food tract. A naturopathic or chiropractic physician can show you a simple technique for keeping that hiatal hernia aligned. Also, you may wish to sleep on your side to avoid sleep time aspiration. (That should help the snoring, too!)

Pain

With most brain-related accidents, the surrounding soft tissue experiences some level of a whiplash incident. With that comes neck and shoulder pain, mid-back pain, low back pain, carpal tunnel trigger to the arms and wrists, and all sorts of other muscular damage. Left untreated, it may compound. (See the chapter "Pain.") It will not resolve on its own. Consider massage therapy.

Survival Energy

The brain is injured, the body is out of whack, and your energy level is unpredictable and relentlessly sapped by chronic physical pain. This could feel like a life-or-death experience, a struggle that makes no sense on a logical level. Just look in the mirror. Aside from the sunglasses and the mismatched clothes, you look perfectly normal. So why does it feel like survival?

It will take a while to lose that "running on empty" feeling. The truth is, you **are** running on empty. Your systems are overwhelmed and overworked, working full-time on the healing process. Your energy supply is in constant doubt. Your brain has gone underground to get fixed. Your body hurts, and the gears are not cooperating with one another.

Is this the end of my life as I know it? Well, yes. At least for a while. But that does not have to be bad news. (See the chapter "New Abilities and New Skills.")

DECEMBER 31, 1993: RECOVERY OF YOUR SKILLS WITHIN TWO YEARS

My doctors told me that my brain would do the healing it was capable of within two years. That I should not expect a lot of continued recovery beyond that two-year time frame. While that may be a workable estimate for them, I continue to recover, develop, progress, enhance, and reclaim function and memory well beyond that guess. Do not let a number frame your recovery. I can and have pointed to specific successes well beyond two years' time. I have decided that I shall continue to reclaim function indefinitely. Happily, this frame of mind is working for me.

Specifically, in the area of physical activity, the progress continues. Having been a very physically active person prior to my accident, a return to my previous level of effort has been a road littered with short bursts, big plans, long walks, inconsistent exercise programs, hikes that were over my head, and a profound feeling of total failure and despair about reclaiming my "power Body." Twenty-five pounds crept onto my frame as those months turned into years.

I questioned my ability to exercise successfully. Must I bid farewell to my beloved outdoors and be content with day hikes, car camping, and modest ski touring? No, my heart shouted, no!

The struggle continued. I knew I had to stick with it. Recommitment to the goal meant dedicating my daily lunch hour four times a week to working out. I joined a health club just three blocks from my office. It was hard to go. Remembering to load the gym bag the night before. Finding clothes to fit. Dreaming of the day I could wear the slinky hot pink tights again.

Daily it is a challenge to go. Pushing through the pain of living a new schedule. Pushing through the emotion of giving priority status to my recovering body. Pushing through the embarrassment of working out next to professional athletes and body fanatics. Remembering that I have my own path to walk, and to stay focused on my personal goals, progress, and triumph.

Staying with it even through the tears rolling down my face walking the treadmill. Tears for no reason I can think of. Tears that insist on flowing. Taking a break in the locker room until the tears stop. Going back out there and finishing the workout.

Acknowledging myself for the courage to show up and the courage to push through the tears and remain focused. I have found a new level of commitment and accomplishment in recovery, and the empowerment to remember I can stick with it consistently. A new level of accomplishment, another rung in the ladder climbed. Another ridge gained.

Paramount for me through all this is the energy and esteem to go back tomorrow. Eighty-five percent of life is just showing up.

Two years is a very short time, given my lifespan. My intention is to continue to heal and expand my brain abilities. It isn't over 'til it's over, and I choose to continue to heal.

Still recovering:

JUNE 4, 1998: MT. RAINIER

This is my third attempt to climb Mt. Rainier. The first attempt since my injury. I spent six months training in the gym almost daily. Lifting weights. Running a mile. Able to run two miles just before the trip. The thrill was in the doing. I made it to the trip. Carrying my own pack. Sunset on Mt. Adams, Mt. St. Helens, and Mt. Hood made it all worthwhile.

DECEMBER 7, 1998: NEVER GIVE UP

Seven and one-half years post-accident I am still recovering vital function. Today is my 49th birthday. I celebrate reclaiming a higher level of cognitive energy and intellectual acuity, due, I am convinced, to my foray into behavioral optometry.

Before I entered vision therapy, I had reached a rehab plateau that lasted about 4 years. Now I feel launched into a realm of reclaimed skills, energy, and creativity that I thought impossible to regain. You never know what new turn in the road will bring you to your next layer of healing. I am thrilled, and yes it is hard work. Happy birthday to me!

Summary

Remember that your body is totally overwhelmed. This is a time to be gentle, nurturing, and quiet with yourself. As you allow your systems to regain their equilibrium, the desensitization will continue and the symptoms should continue to abate. Other chapters will guide you to activities and behaviors that may enhance your progress.

28

Vision

The eyes are the mirror to the soul. So, too, are they the mirror to the brain. So sensitive is the nervous system that stress in the injured brain is reflected in the ability of the eyes to function. Blind spots, fuzzy spots, shower curtain spots, spots from being in lit rooms, and general blurred vision indicate the amount of visual pressure and mental confusion caused by using your eyes in the presence of a brain injury. The central issues here are diffuse axonal stretching of nerve cells in the cranium, optic nerve damage, and optic pathway damage within the central nervous system.

This chapter deals with the vision issues that may be associated with a mild brain injury and suggested therapies for resolution. Vision therapy is offered by behavioral optometrists.

FEBRUARY 7, 1992

My eyes are blurred again. Defocused. Unable to read well or see the words in a book or newspaper.

At first not being able to read seemed a part of the injury. And my attention span and comprehension factors made it just as well. Even if I read, content retention failed. Watching TV had about the same effect. Nice to pass the time. Soaps or CNN, no real difference. Mostly just a matter of taste and pride that I stuck to CNN, Oprah, and old movies.

Even the hematologist asked me about soap operas. I admitted to preferring to watch the birds in my blooming catalpa tree. I'd try to read. Paying the bills worked, occasionally reading legal documents, get well cards, and the funnies. But the rest would blur after a bit.

Visual Disturbances

Visual disturbances such as blind spots, "anonymous informer" spots (I call them mice), fluorescent light spots, eyestrain from computer terminals and televisions, and mental confusion from different light sources are common after mild brain injury. Partial blindness, and even temporary blindness (what I call eye shutdown), is common. Scary, but common.

Your glasses' prescription may change. You may need glasses, temporarily or permanently, for the first time. Photophobia, or sensitivity to light, is common. Sunglasses will help both indoors and outdoors. Light sensitivity can produce an eye headache or a face headache. Consider eliminating fluorescent lighting from your environment.

Vision and Cognition

Your eyes are connected directly to your brain. In fact, the eyes and brain are actually made from the same neural layer in the fetus. What you see and how you recognize what you see—cognition—may be slowed or hampered. For instance, you may read a book passage or the funnies. Five seconds later you may not be able to relate what you read to others or even to yourself. This takes tremendous energy you may not have at your disposal.

MAY 6, 1993

The time lapse between what I see and how I relate to it, then shifting or turning my head or eyes to something new, feels like a time machine. Moving my head to focus my eyes on a new subject creates a time distortion that makes me feel unconnected as I transfer my focus from A to B.

Tasks as "simple" as driving, consulting the rearview mirror, then returning to the front driving view is an eye and brain journey to three places, with time lapses at intervals. The transition is fragmented, like still photos projected before me, with only the film progression noise of the camera missing. Mechanical and outside my control.

Consequently, glass has been broken and fingers have been cut. There have been near misses in the car. People are bumped into. Keyboard strokes are mooshed, food misses the refrigerator shelf and smashes to the floor. Compost jackknifes off the bucket rim and decorates the kitchen wall. Life has become very messy.

But I Have to Use My Eyes!

Yes, using the eyes is vital in our visual culture. Literacy is high, and most of our activities are vision based. When vision goes on the fritz, there is definitely trouble.

What's Wrong?

With mild brain injury, the eyes may change shape and the muscles around the eyes may not work efficiently. Your eyeballs may not be working as a team focused on the same subject. So your "visual perceptual speed," or the ability of your eyes to move in order to perceive what is out there, is changed. Your eyes cannot perform their job like they used to. Therefore, your brain cannot report what your eyes see as accurately or as quickly as before. Your vision is altered.

The Binocular Thing

The main issue with post brain trauma binocular vision is that the eyes have trouble working together. Symptoms of this condition, when they were not experienced before the accident, may include

- Headaches, eye and face headaches, and facial tension

- Blurry vision when looking far away

- Blurry vision when looking close up

- Blurry vision when changing focus from far to near or near to far

- Dizziness or nausea when changing focus or aim

- Double vision—seeing two of something

- Stable objects appear to move

○   Staring behavior—looking off into space, daydreaming

○   Poor vision memory—not remembering where you last saw the keys

○   Poor concentration or attention span

○   Discomfort when reading, sewing, drawing, or using the computer

○   Problems with balance, coordination, or posture

○   Light sensitivity, both to brightness and to rapid changes from one to the other

Remember, it's not that the eyes don't work, rather, that they don't remember how to work together. The eyes must be retrained to work together again. In a way, they are like a computer. All the settings have been erased. You can no longer "press any key to continue." All the data must be re-input and integrated again. The relationship of all the information must be rebuilt again. Your eyes need treatment with a behavioral optometrist. Get an appointment.

Losing Your Place

Objects seem to move. You can lose your place on the page while reading. You can lose your place in traffic while driving (this is more dangerous). Your eyes can converge insufficiently. Your eyes can under aim. You can see things out of the corner of your eye that do not exist (anonymous informer).

Energy

It takes energy to aim the eyes together, and it takes energy to look. If you use up your energy by seeing, there is less left for the brain to process what you see and to retain the information. The more energy you need for input, the less is left for through-put. In fact, vision takes more energy than most other physical activities. Basically, your eyes suck energy like a toaster.

Accommodation

Focus, or accommodation, is messed up with a mild brain injury. It becomes hard to see close up, to "focus." And, if you aren't already 40 years old and experiencing presbyopia (difficulty seeing near objects either with distance glasses for nearsightedness or in general), brain injury can hasten that process. Some days your eyes may be too stressed for you to see well and, consequently, to think efficiently.

Field Defect

Missing pieces of the vision field are called "field defects." You may be missing a vision quadrant or a half field. Blind spots or peripheral vision defects may be evident as well.

Driving

"Convergence insufficiency" is particularly noticeable while driving, and it carries more consequences. You may find that you cannot drive faster than 25 MPH. This appears to be a breakthrough speed in the recovery of your binocular strength. Do not drive until you are able to see and react with sufficient cognitive speed and energy. Let the behavioral optometrist and the driving school be the judge of that.

The Effects of Medications

Fully investigate the effects of any medication you are taking during this time. Some medications exacerbate vision issues. Antihistamines will dry your eyes and mouth. Antidepressants and other brain-injury medications may affect focus and acuity. Medications may also have an effect on your net gain in therapy. Know what you are taking, and weigh the results versus the side effects once you understand them.

The Eye Is Not a Camera

The statement that the eye is a camera is a metaphor, not a physiologic reality. Many of your visual skills originate in the midbrain. The injury to the brain affects your eyes at the level of the cell bodies of your brain. Diffuse axonal stretching, sheering, or pulling of the nerve connectors and their surrounding soft tissue may occur in the midbrain, and will not show up on a CT scan or an MRI.

The job of the midbrain is to connect reflex (primitive, old) brain information to the cerebral (new) brain. It is the pathways between these areas from which visual skills originate.

The optic nerve, the nerve from the pupil, and most extraocular muscles are connected to the midbrain. The oculomotor nerve controls three of the six muscles for each eye, and the trochlear and abducens nerves each control one extraocular muscle in each eye. They all originate in the midbrain. In addition, the ability to focus and the pupils are also affected by the sympathetic and the parasympathetic nervous systems. Plainly, the eyes are hardwired into the brain. When you experience a mild brain injury, your eyesight will likely be involved.

What to Do

Dizziness and nausea can keep most folks grounded, so it is a good place to start. First of all, understand that these symptoms are reasonable for the moment. Your vision therapist may have a treatment plan. I further suggest that you move slowly, but move. Live through the situation. Push gently through. Function in spite of it, breathing deeply and purposefully. Most dizziness and nausea will moderate with this approach.

To rest your eyes successfully, sit or lie down in a quiet, dimly lit room. Rub your hands together until your palms are warm. Place your warm palms over your closed eyes, and hold the position for up to 15 minutes.

The acupressure charts at the end of this chapter will offer you pressure points you can gently press for help in relaxing the face and resting the eyes.

Visualization, cross-crawling behaviors, and various educational kinesiology positions are also helpful.

Eye Lights

Eye Lights are a very effective vision therapy, stimulating the brain and balancing visual and cognitive function. They fit like sunglasses, have various colored shields (depending upon the color your practitioner deems appropriate), and include little flashing lights that stimulate the brain at timed intervals. I obtained mine from my chiropractic neurologist.

Other Tools

The Tibetan Eye Chart on page 226 will also assist you in retraining your eye muscles to work together. To use the chart, hang it on the wall at eye level. You may wish to copy this chart or purchase a separate Tibetan Eye Chart at a bookstore that specializes in holistic reading material. Stand close, or at the point where it is in good focus. First with both eyes, visually trace the outline of the chart, first clockwise, then counterclockwise. Then, covering one eye with your hand (not closing one eye, that does not work), then the other, repeat the procedure.

Remember to keep breathing and to blink naturally. Practice for a few minutes at a time, so that your eye muscle strength is slowly and steadily increased. Avoid further eye strain. Proceed slowly and gently.

Glasses

You may need new glasses and new sunglasses. You may find that sunglasses with certain color filters protect your eyes from light better than do others. Compare the lens-color choices at the opticians by taking them outside to test in daylight. Another product, color therapy glasses, is available in natural food stores and alternative health and book stores offering different color choices. One particular color may give you more relief from eye fatigue, or allow you to read for longer periods of time. (Test these colors outdoors also, to avoid the intrusion of fluorescent lights from the store.)

Reading

Reading with colored glasses may assist you as well, since many paper surfaces glare, or reflect the light in your environment and cause eye fatigue. This book is printed on paper meant to minimize glare. You may have also noticed that this book uses a slightly larger typeface, and more generous spacing. These features were chosen to make reading this book as comfortable for your eyes as possible.

Here's a Neat Trick

One way to decide if your eyes are working well together is to gather up two bathroom scales. Set them side by side. Weigh yourself on each one, and determine that they are synchronized. Now, place them side by side. Put one foot on each scale. Look straight ahead and have a helper look at the scales to report the results.

If your eyes are working well, the amounts will be identical. If the amounts are unequal, consider vision therapy.

Summary

Your eyes are directly connected to your brain. Be gentle with them. *(Special thanks.[7])*

Acupressure Exercise 1.

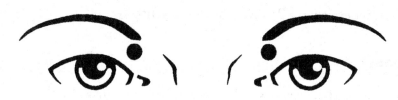

Close your eyes, sit quietly and relax. Place your thumbs in the position indicated by the dots on the diagram above. These dots represent what are known as the Tian Ying points. Your fingers should gently rest on your forehead. Now alternate periods of firm pressure up and in on the Tian Ying points, with periods of relaxation with the thumbs simply resting on the points. Each period should last for about one second. Press, release, press, release, etc. Continue for about two minutes. Make sure you are not pressing against the eyeball.

Acupressure Exercise 2.

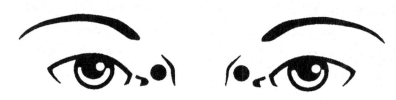

With your eyes closed, use your thumb and forefinger to massage the bridge of your nose, as indicated in the diagram above. Firmly press, then squeeze with a forward motion, to stimulate what is known in acupressure as the Fu Jing Ming points. Do not pinch the skin on your nose. Now release the pressure.

Now press again. Now release. Alternate one second of pressure with one second of relaxation, for about 30 seconds. Press, release, press, release, press, release, etc. Now change hands and do another 30 seconds of the exercise.

Acupressure Exercise 3.

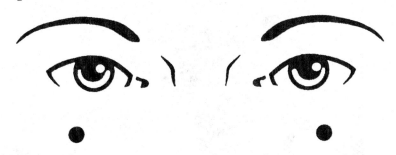

Place two fingers on the Si Bai points located on the crest of the cheekbones, as shown above. Close your eyes. Now gently press against the cheekbones, and move your fingers in a circular motion-slowly pulling your facial muscles as far as they will go. This will make your face feel as if it were made of Jell-O. Make 30 slow circles in one direction, then 30 in the opposite direction.

Acupressure Exercise 4.

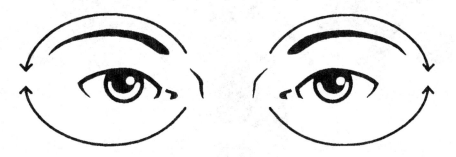

Position your index fingers on the upper dots. Firmly stroke your eyebrows using the flat part between the first and second joints of your index fingers, as indicated by the upper arrow. Now firmly stroke below your eyes with your index fingers, as indicated by the lower arrow. Make alternate strokes between the eyebrows and below the eyes, spending about one second on each stroke, for a total of one minute: Upper, lower, upper, lower, upper, lower, etc...

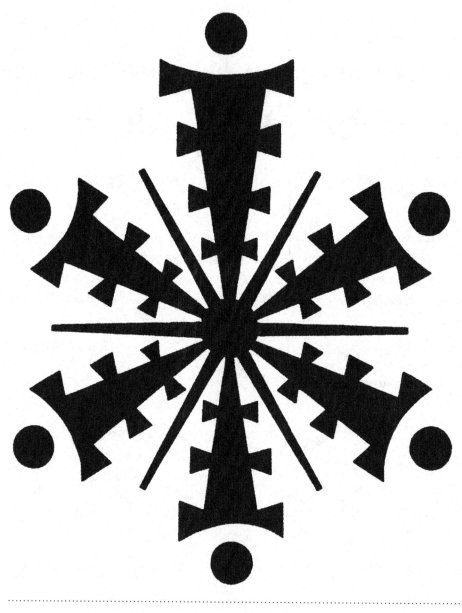

Tibetan Eye Chart

29

Pain and Chronic Pain Management

With a brainlash or other movement accident, your brain probably was not the only part of you that sustained an injury. Soft tissue injuries generally accompany a whiplash-like accident. By "soft tissue" I mean muscle, fascia and connective tissue such as tendons and ligaments. The muscles of the neck, face, jaw, shoulders, arms, and midback are often affected when the brain is injured.

Pain from headache, clenching of the jaw, temporal mandibular joint syndrome (TMJ), neck ache, stiffness in the shoulders, and even carpal tunnel syndrome triggered from neck injury are a few of the possible sources of nagging pain. Left untreated, these conditions can cause long-term, chronic symptoms such as fibromyalgia, headaches, chronic fatigue, immune system weakening, and teeth clenching with subsequent dental damage.

Pay attention to your "pain." This chapter will discuss the soft tissue injuries associated with brain injury and will suggest soft tissue therapies that may be appropriate for your situation.

Hypochondria Disclaimer

You may or may not experience any of the following pain symptoms. Soft tissue pain may accompany brain injury, but it is not a requirement. This pain may or may not set in quickly. The nature of soft tissue injury is such that it may take days, weeks, and in some cases months to set in. Do not rule your pain in or out because of the time factor. Pay attention to any persistent pain you experience. Report it to your healthcare providers, and journal it.

Pain Issues

If your head has been lashed, jostled, twisted, abruptly moved, or intersected with the earth at an unpleasant angle, you also are likely to have experienced soft tissue injury. Physical pain from soft tissue injury may include a low-grade persistent headache;, neck pain; a tight jaw; a tight face; jaw and teeth clenching at night; an involuntary forced smile; tinnitus (ringing in the ears); tight scalp; headache; upper back or shoulder stiffness; radiating pain of the arm and hand; tingling fingers; swollen joints; tight breathing; poor digestion; frequent choking on food, water, or saliva; eye pain, eye headache, or eye twitching; hunched shoulders (shoulders up to your ears), or any combination of these.

Long-term or untreated effects of these pains may result in midback and low-back pain, temporal mandibular joint syndrome, carpal tunnel syndrome, intractable headache, and permanent dental damage. Chronic myofacial pain may be avoided with early and appropriate intervention but not in all cases. Fibromyalgia is rheumatic in nature, and your trauma may also trigger this condition.

None of this sounds like any fun. The key is to identify your pain early and seek appropriate and effective therapy immediately. Suffering is not necessary. Pain will not get better on its own. If you ignore it, it won't go away. If you are getting aches and pains, seek soft tissue therapy. Just "dealing" with your pain will consume stamina and prolong your overall recovery.

Soft Tissue Therapies

Appropriate treatment for your pain depends upon what works for you. The Western model includes osteopathy, physiatry, physical therapy, and walking. The holistic model includes massage and various other therapies, listed below. How you and your healthcare providers design and select your course of treatment is vital to a positive outcome for you.

Massage Therapy

You may benefit from clinical massage therapy. Massage works to benefit the soft tissues involved in your injury, improving circulation to the injured areas. Massage also stimulates the brain by reminding the muscles of their proper function. Your brain benefits by this external modeling. Massage is soothing, allowing you to relax and breathe more easily. Massage is restorative and therapeutic to soft tissue.

Passive Therapies

There are drug-free, effective therapies that offer the muscles and the brain relief from pain and subliminal patterning. The health practitioner assists the brain to re-align its internal energies with the soft tissue and to repair pathways or find new satisfactory pathways to your stored knowledge. Hypnotherapy, creative imagery, guided imagery, and "mindfulness" all assist in this repair of brain paths. (See the chapter "Retrain Your Brain" for scripts called "The Phone Company Exercise," "Office Manager Exercise," and "The Hall of Answers.")

Treating High Levels of Pain

Some subtle energy therapies are indicated and beneficial for extremely painful or chronically painful conditions. Those modalities generally include cranial-sacral therapy, polarity therapy, acupressure, acupuncture, gentle osteopathy, activator chiropractic, Feldenkreis movement, Reiki, gentle Shiatsu, and Aston patterning. For deeper soft tissue work, you may also want to consider neuromuscular therapy, connective tissue massage, Rolfing, chiropractic, and craniosacral osteopathy.

Active Therapies

Active therapies are those that require your participation. Chief among them are walking, dance, yoga, cross-crawling, Pilates exercise, weaving and other arts, and listening to Mozart. Engage in activities you enjoy. They will help you remember what you know. Watch *Jeopardy, Wheel of Fortune, Family Feud,* and *the Discovery Channel.* Watch while others play *Trivial Pursuit, Scrabble,* or *Pictionary.* Old movies and cartoons from your childhood will refresh your memory.

External Modalities

These therapy alternatives will provide you with external patterning models. Experiencing them can reduce pain and offer your brain reminder information. (See "Medical Therapies.")

WALKING   Never underestimate the power of walking. Because walking involves a gentle, rhythmic motion that is repeated over and over, your body becomes more limber during a walk. Simple walking relieves many kinds of aches and pains. Walk every day, whether a few blocks or a few miles. Walking works.

JOURNAL IT   Write down your therapy journey. Keep track of what worked, when, and in what combinations. Learn from the journal.

THERAPEUTIC HORSEBACK RIDING   The latest in brain reeducation therapies is therapeutic horseback riding. Therapeutic riding is designed with the use of gentle horses and trained therapists, and results are impressive. In a nutshell, slow rhythmic horse riding subtly reeducates the core of the central nervous system. The gentle swaying of the animal, and the need for the rider to shift weight one side to the other, appears to accomplish a cross-crawl function. Reports of improvement center around increased mental capacity, reduced physical pain, and improved speech.

The Pain Map

The Seattle Chapter of the Brain Injury Association offers a most complete and informative discussion of pain. I highly recommend their website: ***www.headinjury.com.*** Look for the Pain Map section. Their information and links are helpful and thorough in scope. (See "Resources" for more info.)

Summary

There are many drug-free alternatives to treating soft tissue pain cycles. Remember that this part of your healing process carries with it the recovery aspects of progress, plateau, and refueling. Remain valiant as you venture through the labyrinth. Remember that developing new physical habits demands effort. Do your best every day.

30

Relapse

Failure. Relapse feels like complete and utter failure. You were doing really well. Had a couple of "good brain days" in a row. The curtain had finally lifted. You were sure you'd attained the final breakthrough. You've worked hard for that feeling. Then, CRASH. Brain shuts off. The world stops. You feel like you did something wrong. It feels like you have to start all over again, from the very beginning.

This chapter discusses setbacks, or what appear to you as setbacks. The healing process has a special ebb and flow. Understanding this will help you accept and cooperate with relapse sessions. We will discuss vulnerability, self-care, and control as the healing process continues.

No Dwelling on the Negative

We shall have none of that. Relapse, healing rest, or refueling is a natural part of the process of recovery. It may not be the fun part, but it is a sure sign of recovery.

Relapse and Vulnerability

For a while there, you really thought you were getting better. Then, WHAM. Slam dunk, back to the pain of recovery and the ugly reminders that you have a long way to go. From feeling tall to feeling small and defenseless in one moment is a disconcerting betrayal. Your life may be plunged back to the couch. You remain fragile.

You are unceremoniously reminded of your vulnerability. Memories of how great last week was swamp your thoughts. You hang onto that rope as it slips through your fingers. Enforced rest has returned.

You remember enforced rest. It is your friend. You are back to the basics. Not "square one" exactly, but all the fundamentals apply.

The Healing Process Chart

Here's the chart that will graphically demonstrate the healing process. Notice how there are three stages in each segment of the process. Focus on the progress section. This is how your body feels when working well. Notice the plateau process. This is a maintaining time, when you cruise. Now see the refueling process, when you backslide and experience healing rest.

Notice most especially that the cumulative effect works its way UP, toward continued improvement. This is the result of linking all the segments together. Like a dance that goes "two steps forward, one step to the side, one step backward," you will eventually get across the dance floor. The cumulative effect is positive and is termed "integration of gain."

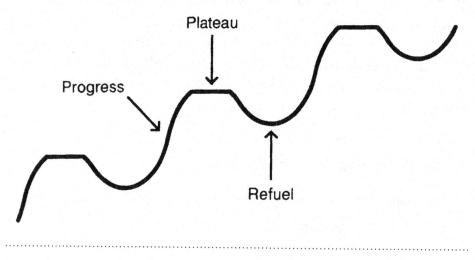

Integration of Gain (The Healing Process)

Setbacks Are a Part of the Deal

Reframe your setback as a dynamic part of the process of healing. Just as you cannot drive across country without buying gas every now and then, so too with your recovery. You gotta buy gas. And you gotta stop the engine first. Says so right on the sign.

Ambushed Again

Relapse can certainly feel like failure, there is no doubt about that. It feels as if you have to start all over again. That can be devastating to self-esteem and emotionally painful. And because it can feel like an ambush, you may think you are out of control again.

You Remain in Control

You will realize that you remain in control when you discover that this is a process and understand the necessity for enforced rest. Conscious cooperation with the healing graph keeps you in the driver's seat. Once you understand the need for each step, suddenly you realize your positive participation in the process returns control of your emotions and your behavior choices. That's better.

This refueling time is as integral as the progress and plateau times. Keep a positive attitude about the whole process, and remain in control. No need to feel fragile anymore. Knowledge is power! You are doing great! Gain is a three-step process.

NOVEMBER 23, 1992

I can't tell whether this missing piece is "good" or "bad." The sensitivity barrier seems weakened. I can't seem to fend off unkindly remarks or random orneriness from others. The protective shield is gone. The tears flow more easily and steadily at the slightest advance. Is that good? A threat? Just exhausting?

Three days ago my brain plunged backward, what seemed a year into deep fuzzy unconnectedness, as if someone had turned the screwdriver the wrong direction, then did it again, thinking it would help.

The flashback memory of all the struggle—pain—isolation—nonproductivity—stagnation and the sense of having to start all over *again* brought sobs and tears that would not stop. Oh no—I'd slipped backward, really far, this time. All that work, all that effort, for what? A surprise relapse? Great! Could this happen *again* at any time? For no apparent reason?

Then a small voice said, "Hook up the two sides of the brain again, just like you used to. Visualize the phone company workers on each side of the corpus callosum connecting wires to each other through the wall; hook up some wires."

Was this a setback, or just the next layer of the onion peeling away, unannounced? I couldn't stay this way forever. I had been subpoenaed to a deposition. My brain *had* to work tomorrow. This wasn't funny. I willed my brain to reconnect. I remained dull, flat all day. Nothing lifted. I wandered around the house, engaging in repetitive uninteresting tasks. The fuzz was back. Would this possibility never subside?

Next week is my birthday. I will be 43. I announce it proudly, my graying hair bouncing, lively above the twinkle in my eyes. One and a half years old since my brush with death.

This new me is glad—nay, grateful—to be here and to be celebrating. It's harder when the new pieces of me act up, or act out, or run low on fuel. Yes, I want to be alive. Why do I feel damaged today? My eyes won't read, my smile is painted on. I want to sit and stare. There's an engagement ring on my long and slender finger. Size 5. A single blue sapphire glistens on two golden wings. It's been there only a few days now. It sways, moving about as my hand makes its way through the day, in and out of pockets, gloves, water, and paper shuffling.

This man loves me. Holds me in his heart just as he held my hand, kneeling in the snow, to ask if the ring might be worn on my hand. A simple "Yes, I will" came from my heart and bounced off the fir trees and shimmer of uncut powder, making its way to those true blue eyes. "Yes, I will." With tears and hardly a breath of chilled air to draw. Loved. But when my brain shuts off, suddenly the isolation returns and with it the pain of shattered self-esteem. The devastation of another recovery episode. Frustration screams for an end to the torture. Let me think. Let me live. Let me be.

Slinking slower than gray shadows of later sunset, the internal cloud hangs low, darkening the horizon, delaying even the moonlight reflecting recognition behind my glasses. All I wanted to do was read the newspaper.

Understand the Process and Let Yourself Heal

There is truly a sense of peace when this portion of the healing is understood. In the shrink biz, we call it "letting go," or surrendering. I wrote a poem.

The Gift of Moving Toward the Heart

> The day that survival is no longer the question
> Is the day one may purely and effortlessly
> Live from the heart.
>
> The effort involved
> In watching over the shoulder
> Takes all the reserves and more.
>
> When survival is no longer the question,
> Peace at heart becomes
> The answer.

Summary

Refueling or healing rest are vital activities to express the concept of what may feel like a relapse. Understanding integration of gain will ease you through those painful times. Journal your progress. Relapse days are perfect days to read about your progress and to remember how far you have come. Look forward to the progress ahead. Remember, all parts of the process in cooperation and balance render a positive upward result. Keep your eye on the prize.

31

Medical Therapies

Aside from the opportunities offered by the Western medical model for the rehabilitation of mild brain injury, numerous additional external modalities have been identified as assisting in recovery. Please review the ***medical disclaimer*** on the copyright page before proceeding.

This chapter stresses personal responsibility for recovery. The following therapies are suggested in addition to your physician-directed care. The efforts of a therapeutic team are optimal. The movable feast of effective therapies is yours to explore, evaluate for effectiveness, and experience.

Not all listed therapies may be available in your area. Not all of these suggested therapies may be appropriate for you. Certain combinations may work better for you than do others. Personal awareness and journaling will assist you in your selection decisions and each modality's effectiveness in your case.

This chapter will be most effective once you have resolved any feelings of victimization that accompany you to this point. Blame, excuses, whining, or secondary gain are not honest and will hinder or delay your healing process. Life is not fair. Life is simply life. This is your life and here is the next step.

Journal what you try. Record what you observe. Pay attention to results.

Western Medical Model

Modern medicine has much to offer, especially in areas that directly apply to intervention medicine. To date, however, this model offers little that treats the mildly brain injured. Without an external bump on the head, the Western model holds no strong belief that measurable or diagnosable internal damage has occurred. The Western model focuses on the severely brain-injured patient and applies intervention medicine as appropriate. You don't need surgery. Your symptoms don't show up on the bar graph.

A few therapies within this model do apply to mild brain injury and are covered by your insurance company. Do not overlook these areas of opportunity, as they can be most beneficial to your recovery. The key here is proper diagnosis and referral by prescription to these therapies. Generally, the areas include physical therapy, occupational therapy, neurology, ophthalmology, behavioral optometry, osteopathy, physiatry, psychiatry, and clinical psychotherapy. If your insurance plan includes the use of these applications, by all means benefit from them.

Holistic Medical Model

More contemporary insurance companies are seeing the wisdom of preventive medical modalities, and their benefits focus on maintaining optimal health. When intervention is necessary, it may then be less invasive or costly. Generally, those modalities covered may include chiropractic, massage, nutrition, exercise, acupuncture, herbal remedies, homeopathy, and a score of other options, often at the discretion of the insurer.

Optional Holistic Health Model

Medical models from many cultures on our planet are being shared, practiced, and promoted in Western culture. They include traditional Chinese, Tibetan, Indian, Native American, Japanese, and other long-standing medical systems. The beneficial aspects of these systems are many and varied and are best explored with the assistance of a qualified practitioner.

The Western counterculture movement of the 60's created a polyglot of seemingly unconnected health belief systems, which have tended to be viewed as hippie or granola-head medicine. With lots of jokes about the wonders of tofu, sprouts, and carrot juice, this early attempt at exploring the value of alternative medical models has brought us slowly but surely to an era of holistic medicine. The good news is, the productive and successful modalities evolved from that era have moved into the complementary medical model and are available for your exploration.

Subtle Energy Medicine

The "alternative medicine" culture, also known as Complementary Medicine, has evolved into a research-based, scientifically grounded body of knowledge known as subtle energy medicine. Hard science, such as quantum physics, is being applied to traditional medical models with sound research and success. And, as with the Western model, it works whether or not you believe in it.

This chapter will highlight those facets of the Western model that apply to your recovery process. We will further explore those aspects of alternative or subtle energy medicine that may also enhance your recovery process. The key to your success in choosing modalities that are appropriate for you is to take personal responsibility for your recovery. When you assume that position, you can ask yourself if a therapy feels appropriate, if it appears to be working, if you are ready for it, and when you wish to end it. Journaling enhances your ability to evaluate and decide.

Medical Self-Responsibility

So, what to do? Medical self-responsibility means, plainly, that you are responsible for your own recovery. No one is as passionate about your recovery as you are. You hold the most vested interest in the outcome.

There are modalities that can help you to one extent or another, depending upon your situation and the severity of your condition. Your participation is key. Yes, this accident happened to you. No, you did not ask for it. No, it may not have been your fault. No, the other guy cannot be eternally responsible for you. No, your insurance company may not pay for alternative therapies, let alone the contractual treatments.

You have a life to heal and live. You can be stuck in blame, or you can get on with the task at hand: healing your brain, lifting your depression and getting on with life. It will not be pretty. It will take time. You won't be the same person you were before. Whining or healing: which do you prefer?

Release the Victim Mentality

Of course, it is a drag to have a brain injury. Tell me about it. Self-pity can be a part of the process, too, as long as you intend to linger briefly, then move through and beyond it.

There is no self-respect or self-responsibility in the "secondary gain" of the victim mentality. When you are ready to let go of the source of your circumstances and move toward restoring your health, then this chapter is for you.

Transporting blame, excuses, and pity into this chapter will surely slow you down. It gets in the way. The truth is no excuse. It's just the truth.

Record Your Therapy

Ultimately, you are the judge of whether or not a therapy is working for you. What are the expected results? Are you moving toward them? What is your role in ensuring the success of the therapy? Are there follow-up activities? Are you capable of participating in them at this time? What support will assist your success?

Pay attention to what you try, and in what combinations and intervals. Your personal "recovery cocktail" will be different from anyone else's. Not only that, you may discover that your needs change within the "cocktail." For me, it seems like the target moves and I have to keep adjusting, fine-tuning, and rearranging the therapy so that the efficiency remains focused.

Notice what works, and for how long. For instance, if I have a massage, then my muscles may feel good for two days. If I have a massage followed by a hot tub, the muscles may feel good for three days. If I continue this treatment schedule, eventually I can stretch the massage frequency to every four days, then five, etc.

Keep track of what works, in what combination, for how long, and for how many sessions. Note time of day, meals eaten, body regularity, water intake. If this all sounds overwhelming, ask for help from your support mentor in keeping track and in analyzing what you have noticed. Use the journal notebook format found in the "Journaling" chapter.

Keep the receipts or pay by check for all therapy, keeping short notes to back up your experience. You may spend enough money (and drive enough miles) on medical therapies to itemize the deduction on your tax return. Your records will assist you in tracking those expenditures.

Medical Tax Deduction

Your insurance company may not cover these therapies, but you may be able to deduct the medical expenditures from your income tax if they meet the financial criteria. Consult your accountant for the rules. (You may discover that you can deduct not only the therapy costs, but also your travel mileage. Ask your accountant how to best track this.)

External Modalities

This section focuses on the externally applied therapies. By that, I mean suggested therapies experienced from outside your body, such as massage or chiropractic. Internal modalities will be discussed in the "Nutrition" chapter and will describe those therapies that take place inside your body, such as food, vitamins, and herbs. As with either approach, beware practitioners who try to "keep you for themselves" and tell you that their therapy is the only true therapy that will garner results.

The following external modalities are presented for your consideration. Each brain-injured person responds to different therapies in different ways and for different reasons. It is your responsibility to decide whether a particular therapy is appropriate, useful, or necessary. As with any opportunity, just because it exists does not mean it has your name on it. Not all known therapies are listed here. If I have forgotten to list one, remember, I have a brain injury, too. Suggest that I add it to the book!

JANUARY 22, 1993: SUBTLE ENERGIES, OR ALL THE THERAPIES YOUR INSURANCE COMPANY REJECTS

After the accident, I spent six days in the hospital, administering Demerol to myself and gradually regaining a sense of place.

Within two or three days, as soon as the tubes were out, I began to take Rescue Remedy and Goldenseal/Echinacea extract. But even before that, I had my Walkman and played the soundtracks of "Out of Africa" and "Man from Snowy River" over and over and over again as I visualized sewing up my incision, which was a life-saving slice from cleavage to navel.

Organic chicken broth, mango ice cream, and fresh orange juice. Nectar of the Gods. Fresh food smuggled in. My house mate played Hacky-sack with the dreaded red hospital Jell-o. Once home, a steady diet of spinach, red meat three times a day, and all the milk and iron pills I could stand. I had two liters of blood to grow.

It was only after the anemia subsided that I began to suspect more problems. Three or four months later, still no attention span. Blind spots in my eyes. Hard to read. Very low comprehension. Watching "Jeopardy," knowing the answers, knowing I knew the answers, unable to blurt them out.

There is something wrong here. But what is it? After the initial recognition of cranial deficit and the subsequent "tests," I decided to try unconventional, subtle energy therapies. With a PhD in holistic health, I had a few ideas of my own.

So I consulted friends and colleagues in various fields, read when my eyes would work, and did what I could remember to do. Although the order and frequency of many of these categories escapes me, as I tried several before I could write, and didn't think to record them (it didn't seem like an organized series at the time) they all seemed valuable. Some singly, some in combos.

Not cast in stone, as no therapies are cure-alls or designated for all people in all cases. I submit them for your consideration of their benefit to me. And suspect that they worked with each other synergistically. The data are skimpy, but the results in some cases were obvious, subtle in others.

Acupuncture

Acupuncture operates on the electrical patterns of the body and is used to balance energy. Stimulating selected points on the head and face energized my thinking, sometimes cleared my vision and released the tension in my face. Clenching developed and temporomandibular joint syndrome from oral stress were a factor also. Acupuncture also speeded the cosmetic healing of my scar, so I had external evidence that the process was effective. There were also times when the treatment would overstimulate my brain and make me anxious and confused. Be sure to tell your practitioner, as this can be changed. Feedback is vital here. Honor the wisdom in your body. Communicate with your practitioner.

ElectroAcupoint® Therapy, the latest in pain-free acupuncture technology, employs a very sensitive electronic, handheld sensor applied to the skin. This sensor is capable of detecting the electrical low-impedance condition of a trigger point or acupuncture point that is malfunctioning and causing a loss of balance between the muscles and the nervous system. ElectroAcupoint® Therapy treats the trigger points and acupuncture points without using needles, and the stimulation sensation is mild. I found this method of therapy much more relaxing and less painful than traditional acupuncture. (Available for purchase on the web.)

Aston Patterning®

Aston Patterning is, in my opinion, one of the most effective and therapeutically based bodywork techniques available. Many registered physical therapists are also Aston Patterners. This is a hands-on therapy that includes stretching and also movement education, ergonomics, and fitness training to support the work and integrate changes in your body's function. Aston Patterning reminds your body of its natural functioning state.

Most intriguing for me is how this therapy "unwinds" an injury. Dealing with the mechanism of injury as the road map, it works with the soft tissue in a massage/physical therapy manner to undo the impact of an accident. Movement is restored, especially when trauma is involved. I am very impressed with this painless therapeutic application of bodywork.

Astrology

This is an ancient tool that has been studied for thousand of years and used in countless cultures, East and West. Finding out your chart for the day of your accident will give you another understanding of your situation. My accident day chart revealed an incredible amount of personal and professional change, a shift in emphasis to more spiritually focused work, a definite notation on publishing, writing and speaking, teaching, and sharing. I consulted this reading one and a half years after the accident and noted that those shifts had indeed taken place. The accident seemed to slam-dunk me in that direction (also indicated), and coincidence is simply a safe stance for the skeptical. Astrology assisted me in making some sense of the event and encouraged me in my pursuit of other avenues of vocation. Believing or not believing is not a function of astrology. The planets and constellations move whether we believe in their relationships, symbologies, or metaphors. Suspend your belief system and simply receive the information. It is another tool of recovery. (P.S. Real astrologers are not weird people in costumes. Shopping around is good. Your horoscope in the paper is recreational and not specific enough.) Further, this modality is most useful when perceived in metaphor, rather than as linear information.

Behavioral Optometry

The therapy branch of the optometry field, behavioral optometry, is a standard Western medicine model for therapy, sadly underadvertised. Eye therapy is taught at optometry school but apparently its appeal is limited. I was never more simultaneously elated and enraged when I discovered not only that could eye therapy give me a tremendous level of intellect and physical energy back, but that it was standard Western medicine and no other physician had recommended it to me. It's practically an underground profession, luckily gaining prominence as successes increase in brain-injury treatment .

Once I began my course of eye therapy, personal miracles and quantum leaps of additional healing began to manifest. This was years after giving up hope for a real chance to get a lot better. Never did I expect results like I received. Within the first six months of therapy, and three glasses prescriptions, amazing changes were evident. My physical stamina improved significantly. My eyesight became stronger and more efficient. My intellectual energy boosted, and creative thinking returned. Critical thinking regenerated. For the first time, I looked back over the last seven years, and I could comprehend my disability and my level of functioning. Physical pain diminished and, with it, about half my chiropractic and massage care frequency. The improvements were phenomenal, and I'm not finished with the therapy. (See "Resources" and also Google: Behavioral Optometry and Neuro-Optometric Rehabilitation Association.)

I must confess, when first I heard about this therapy I just groaned, feeling overwhelmed about one more place to go and be therapized. Now I know it is a cornerstone of my full rehabilitation.

Biofeedback and Neurofeedback

Traditional biofeedback is an effective method of training you to elicit a relaxation response with the use of noninvasive electronic equipment and is readily available through numerous healthcare practitioners. It is indicated for pain management and will introduce you to the influence your trained mind can have over the regulation of your body sensations.

Neurofeedback is the latest in biofeedback therapies, incorporating low-energy electrical stimulation and evaluation. Clinical psychologists and brain-injury therapists offer this successful and cognitively productive modality. (See "Resources.")

Chiropractic

This is a simple, powerful tool that focuses on the mechanical realignment of the skeletal body. It offers dynamic maximum opportunity for the central nervous system to deliver its message. Don't let anyone tell you the skull can't be adjusted. The sutures in the skull are dynamic (they move), yet subtle. It is best to get adjusted after massage, polarity therapy, or cranial-sacral therapy. You are most relaxed then, and the adjustment will hold longer. If you receive care from a chiropractor who doesn't incorporate soft tissue therapies (i.e., massage, physical therapy, cranial-sacral technique), find one who does. The dance between the bones and muscles is a delicately balanced one. Select a chiropractor who understands and practices whole-body chiropractic care.

Chiropractic is one of the most useful therapies I used in my recovery. Chiropractic centers its attention on the central nervous system. Your brain is the boss of the nervous system. Your brain gains support and strength when all the parts of the nervous system are in optimal operating alignment.

There are many different styles of chiropractic. Not only are there the familiar crunch and roll practitioners who make lots of noise when they adjust you, but there are also more gentle, less noisy forms of chiropractic. There are several schools of chiropractic technique. Choose the form of adjusting that best suits your style. This therapy does not have to hurt or scare you with the noises your body makes.

Ask a friend for a referral, or call the local chiropractic association for a referral to the style of doctor that suits your treatment preference. Make sure your chiropractor is familiar with brain injury and believes in balanced holistic care and soft tissue therapy. Many doctors staff massage therapists in their offices.

Chiropractic Neurology

A powerful subspecialty within chiropractic is the chiropractors who are qualified neurologists. They are particularly trained to understand and treat brain injury. Their training guides a brain-based rather than spine-based treatment modality. By evaluating brain function and symmetry of brain output from each side of the brain, the nature of persistent dysfunctional conditions can be better understood and treated. Interactive metronome, brain balance music, colored eye lights, and vestibular balance testing are included and are very helpful. (See "Resources.")

Once I shifted to chiropractic neurology, my overall brain function improved and my treatment frequency reduced significantly.

Cognitive Therapy

There are therapists whose sole focus is retraining the brain. They are known as cognitive therapists and they generally have a masters degree or PhD in psychology. They administer evaluation tests and therapy activities that challenge, stretch, and retrain your brain in the needed areas. Some provide psychotherapy support or have a colleague who provides this adjunct service. Many cognitive therapists also conduct support-group therapy sessions focused on mild brain-injury recovery.

When you join a support group, make sure the goals are defined and focused on recovery. Some groups turn into misdirected whining sessions and may not provide the support for positive progress that you are looking for. Shopping around is good. Make sure you are with your brain-injury peers (only mildly injured.) The needs of the mildly injured are very different from those of the moderately or severely injured. Lumping everyone together will swamp you with unproductive stories and issues.

You may choose to use this text as a study guide for support-group therapy. You may also suggest this book as a text to your cognitive therapist or to friends who are brain injured.

Cranial-Sacral Technique

Based on a theory of "as above, so below," cranial-sacral technique incorporates the subtle aspects of the central nervous system and the fluids, pressures, and pulses in the spinal core or cranial-sacral trunk. It is believed to increase and maximize the physiology of the brain to function at its highest level while encouraging increased flow of cerebral spinal fluid, oxygen, and electrical activity within the central nervous system. This therapy can be subtle and profound. It lunged me forward and also dragged me back to re-experience and clear up old patterns and temporary emotions. It gave me hope, opened up windows in my thinking processes, and made me deal with the devastating parts of brain injury. It further demonstrated to me that my situation was temporary and I was indeed passing through, not passing on, i.e., dead.

The brain can repair itself and, with guidance and encouragement, can reach a greater potential goal than when left to its own devices (i.e., come back in two years and we'll test you again). Most especially, cranial-sacral technique is a powerful *pain reliever*

Lately I have combined cranial-sacral therapy with behavioral optometry and have been remarkably impressed with the results. Because the eyes are wired directly into the brain, the combination of eye therapy and cranial-sacral manipulation has assisted in returning various functions to me that I thought impossible. Most notably, I have regained intellectual and creative ability and a great store of physical energy (previously used to make my misaligned eyes work) and have improved reading skills and comprehension and critical thinking skills. I also let go of headaches and the pain of eye strain. I am thrilled.

Cranial-sacral technique is practiced by osteopathic physicians and massage therapists, among other practitioners. Some are aligned with behavioral optometrists. Insurance support may be available. Check credentials for training at the Upledger Institute. (See Upledger Institute in "Resources.")

Cross-crawling

This term refers to physically crossing the midline with your arms, legs, and eyes. It is a kinesthetic level of rejuvenating the brain and is as easy as touching your right hand to left knee and vice versa, 10 minutes worth every now and then. Cross-crawling is also a term associated with the neurologic reeducation of the entire nervous system, as practiced by cognitive re-education specialists. I personally practiced cross-crawling methods and found success in two notable areas: reduction of severity and frequency of limbic rage episodes and reduced involuntary choking on food or saliva. The techniques are sound, and I recommend them as offering valuable therapy for the rehabilitation of mild brain-injury symptoms. This therapy is based on re-education of the nervous system and the rebuilding of brain function through various physical activities practiced daily.

EMDR

This form of psychotherapy, eye movement desensitization and reprocessing, is highly successful in reframing trauma memory, flashbacks, and repetitive negative thoughts. Offered by psychologists, this effective therapy can soothe memories, soften trauma effects, and offer a calmer more positive outlook to your recovery process.

External Stimuli

External modeling is also known as external stimulation. A good deal of my thinking actually relied on outside stimulation to help me remember what I knew. It was almost as if an external trigger would send a clerk back into the files, to emerge later with a "sure enough, you know that, here it is" smile on her face. As if the data banks were closed but not locked. Only the passwords were missing, and each file had its own. People around me knew them but didn't know I needed them. A double waiting game. "I thought you had it; no, I thought *you* had it."

External stimuli helped me to unlock the stories of my life and recall what I know. It gives the brain new paths to the files. (See "The Phone Company.")

Homeopathy

This is a precise subtle medicine system that focuses on the balance of energy in the body. Homeopathy holds that dysfunction, such as anatomic dysfunction caused by brain injury, shifts the energetic plane of the body. Minute quantities of various remedies are shown to improve symptoms such as depression, vertigo, infection susceptibility, weepiness, sleep disorders, and sexual energy. Because every person's body responds differently to injury and to remedies, working closely with a homeopathic physician may bring about the benefit you desire. Many naturopathic physicians practice homeopathy, as do other healthcare professionals. Your homeopath also needs to know that your depression and lethargy may be sourced differently because of your injury. Seek someone who will take this into account.

Hypnotherapy

This is a form of creative visualization. Guided visualization imaging in a clinical setting puts the brain to work and adds a creative or nonimpaired person to assist in tracing and hooking up brain parts and body parts, discovering what works but is asleep and discovering new routes around dead cells to restore function thought irretrievable. There are uncounted numbers of unemployed brain cells just waiting to be activated. Hypnotherapy is an avenue for locating and enjoining them. If you want them to come out and play, you have to knock on the door and invite them.

Interactive Metronome

This therapeutic modality is effective for improvements in cognitive deficits in attention and concentration, motor planning and sequencing, language processing, and impulsive behavior. Because deficits in executive function mimic ADD and ADHD, this form of therapy can benefit a brain-injured person. Consult your chiropractic neurologist or look for more information at www.interactivemetronome.com.

Laughing

Norman Cousins is still right. Laugh. We watched "Rocky and Bullwinkle" a lot on Saturday mornings. It provided pleasure and repeated a familiar childhood pattern. It reinforced a groove while providing a great time. "Hey Rocky, watch me pull a rabbit out of my hat!"

Because **humor** is a complicated cognitive task, using older, more familiar humor may reestablish that groove more gently than watching the comedy channel. Vintage movies helped to speed my reaction time to humor and to anticipate potentially funny situations. Anticipation and timing are the hallmarks of comedy. Do the Marx Brothers, Three Stooges, Our Gang, Abbott and Costello, Lily Tomlin, and Steve Martin do it for you? Order up a movie and go for it. Laugh your way back to cognitive integrity.

Massage Therapy

This is extremely valuable, reinforcing the natural state of muscles (soft tissue), their correct electrical relationship with the brain, and a consistently repeated pattern of contact and relief. It reinforces the brain and its relationship with the body, re-establishing and repeating information "grooves," as I came to call them, giving the brain a reliable and repeated set of data. A relaxing, reinforcing therapy.

(Massage therapy is a classic example of the strong effects an external modality has in reminding the muscles about the information they hold.

Reminding the body from the outside creates a pathway of remembering that the brain seems to accept. It seems to trigger the brain to say, "Oh yes, I remember this now." More brain doors open with repeated external modalities. Massage therapy is often called by other names, such as neuromuscular re-education, Swedish massage, deep tissue therapy, or medical or clinical massage. Look for credentials from nationally known massage schools. www.amta.com Some states also have licensing.)

Massage therapy for people with brain injuries must be practiced uniquely because the muscles respond differently to treatment than do those of textbook massage clients. Essentially, brain-injury physiology has a muscle response lag time that can be interpreted by the massage therapist as permission to go deeper or work longer. Search for an experienced massage therapist who understands this aspect of undertreating, who won't try to heal you in three sessions, and who sees patience as a part of rehabilitation. Take a copy of this paragraph to your massage session to help explain what you need.

Mozart

Yes, listening to Mozart. Because he was a pure composer who wrote music, not an emotionally destructive, angry, power-projecting, or other ego-extension style. His music is recognized as pristine, unencumbered with suffering or social message. Your brain will love to follow the progressions and can easily absorb the sequences. Audio gymnastics. Splendidly enjoyable mind-calming therapy.

Physical Therapy

Classic physical therapy offers much to the recovery of brain use. Physical therapy focuses on a realistic assessment of the physical effects of brain injury, with treatment to stimulate the areas affected. Physical therapists can test your physical strength and fitness and offer guidelines for restoring your previous fitness levels.

Your right brain is accessed through movement. Physical therapists provide help with perceptual and balance issues. They make use of activities with which you are already familiar and deal with your proprioceptive (movement in space) issues. Physical therapists assist in your body awareness or kinesthetic sense.

Addressing soft tissue evaluation, physical therapy pays attention to the holding patterns in soft tissue that hang on to pain. They watch for compensation patterns (how you move to adjust or avoid pain) and work to correct those patterns.

Physical therapists focus on how you use your body. They apply their abilities to help you change movement patterns and reduce pain. Some physical therapy practices are more focused on brain-injury recovery than are others. Shop around. The good news is that physical therapy is a Western modality that insurance companies are likely to fund. Some physical therapists include craniosacral therapy, Aston Patterning, massage, and other subtle energy applications in their practice.

Pilates Method

This gentle form of exercise and stretching, which builds strength and flexibility quietly and steadily, was a great choice for me in many respects. It is very valuable for the recovery of muscle tone and strength. It requires sequencing and full attention, uses some unusual gym equipment, and can include a private instructor. It makes your brain work, and it acts as a strong external body-movement reinforcement. It reminds your brain how your body moves through space and time.

Mostly, it is a great place for beginners. The motions are simple and gentle, controlled, and safe. There is no bouncing or aerobics. Exercise is encouraged up to, but not including, pain. Rehabilitation-focused Pilates instructors understand the pain factor and support you in your quest for mobility and pain reduction.

Pilates (pronounced: pi-LOT-eze) was the first form of exercise I tried. The simple movements were easy to master because they did not require sequencing at first. No grunting or heavy sweating. Just isolated, controlled movements that protect you from straining your muscles. This form of exercise is very kind to your back. Pilates allowed me to gently and safely return to more active exercising.

I discovered that, while practicing Pilates with an instructor, I was better able to concentrate on the movements of my body with my eyes closed. We experimented with using sunglasses, blindfolds, and just closing the eyes. I found that with my eyes closed I was able to focus and perform the exercises more easily. It seemed as if the strain on my brain was reduced and I was better able to follow through on the instruction. You may wish to explore this aspect but only with a personal instructor present, both for your safety and for the safety of those around you. (Disclaimer: Don't try this at home. Proceed at your own risk. This is my experience, not a recommendation.)

Through behavioral optometry it is clear that the eyes, when working improperly, take a disproportional amount of physical energy to operate. Rehabilitation exercise benefits from eye therapy, adding more energy and reducing fatigue and pain perception.

Polarity Therapy®

This is a body of knowledge synthesized by Dr. Randolph Stone, which holds a key to physical electricity and from which I gained a great deal. Based upon certain subtle electrical fields and looking very eclectic and inclusive of several nontraditional styles, polarity therapy gently realigns the energy of the body, reconnecting unconnected energy flow. It addresses the full balance of body energy, realigning the brain to itself and the rest of the body with which it communicates or presently miscommunicates. It is holistic and centered in balance and reconnects brain and body function, encouraging the body and stimulating it to participate in the healing process. Polarity therapy reduces the effects of trauma and offers the body a break from pain and stress. This form of external modeling, recreating the state of peace and comfort, benefits the brain by offering a success pattern to emulate. Polarity therapy is a certified profession, so check for credentials.

Psychic Healing

This is sometimes called spiritual healing, and it comes in many forms. The healers know who they are. I know the power of this energy because my intuitive abilities have helped many others. In this case, associates simply held me in their thoughts in a "healing way." It is a powerful form of prayer, which simply visualizes the intended patient and holds her in a peaceful, healing, and energizing regard. Enroll your family and friends in this activity as well. Prayer holds its own special value in the healing process and can serve to empower your support group. (If this does not intrigue you, just keep reading. Not all approaches are useful to all people in the same way.)

Psychological Kinesiology

This is a muscle-testing technique that explores your mental or thinking process. One can discover one's state of mind as the brain couches thoughts and beliefs. For instance, say the phrase "I feel safe in the world." Then do a muscle test for a strong or weak response. From there, the therapy responds to track the weak response with more questions. New ideas and suggestions (negotiations) follow to strengthen the response. Fascinating work, especially for the cognitively challenged merging and trying to track the "new logic" in their brains.

Psychotherapy

Serving to discover the manner in which your brain recorded your life history, psychotherapy assists in the reframing of that history so that it can be dealt with, reinterpreted, and lived with in the present. When you have a brain injury, this may not be support that you can use right away.

Psychotherapy for the brain-injured person better centers around understanding and dealing with the present reality of injury, the depression as a result of that injury, and the development of a support system to assist in the healing process.

Delving into the dark reaches of your Self at this time may increase your feelings of being overwhelmed and stressed. Avoid therapy that is not focused on your immediate support needs and daily survival. Avoid being misdiagnosed. Make sure your psychotherapist or clinical psychologist is experienced in brain-injury recovery work. Just say no to psychoanalysis. It is inappropriate because you don't have the energy for it and because it is contraindicated to the goals you presently hold for your recovery.

Quantum Energetics

This is an emerging therapy that focuses on accessing the brain and reminding it of its functions, area by area. I have been impressed with the clarity my brain gains and holds with each treatment I receive. Quantum energetics can stimulate and strengthen your immune system and support your brain in the healing process.

The treatment is external, noninvasive, painless, and effective. Quantum energetics evaluates almost all body systems energetically, so a variety of trauma-related conditions can be addressed. This can include cranial bone trauma, dural trauma, whiplash-type injury, immune system damage, and soft tissue damage.

People with brain injuries report relief from headache, depression, seizures, visual imbalances, cognitive disorders, and speech difficulties. Improved coordination and increased energy levels generally follow. Quantum energetics integrates with and can enhance other therapies such as vision therapy, speech therapy, cranial sacral therapy, and massage therapy. Practitioners of quantum energetic are certified.

Somatic Experiencing

This psychotherapy modality focuses on the reframing and minimizing of the impact of physical trauma and emotional trauma on the body, mind, and emotions. It is a highly effective hybrid of trauma therapies and is practiced by psychologists. Practitioners of Somatic Experiencing are certified.

Visualization

This technique proved very powerful for me. "Crossing the midline" of my body with **cross-crawling** or **educational kinesiology** showed me that my brain messages weren't getting through the brain midline, the switchboard, that is the corpus callosum. There was no cranial cross-over, thus, no sequencing or referencing. My thinking was linear, my brain function was stiff and slow. So I created a visualization for hooking up the right and left brain by pretending that there were phone-company workers on both sides and they were rewiring my brain through the midline. My brain function improved after every visualization session. After a few sessions with that activity, I began to recall information that had been "locked up in file cabinets in my head."

Sometimes I used **visualization** accompanied by music. Just as I sewed my incision back together again to "Out of Africa," so too did I find that the visualization of reconnecting frayed and snapped wires or the search for a new, established but sleeping route could be enhanced with music. Increasing pleasure increases results. The body naturally responds to pleasurable events. Connecting therapy and progress with pleasure creates a setting of effortless effort. Repetition becomes the preferred state. Craving more therapy is the ideal recovery frame of mind. Put it to music!

Yoga

Practicing yoga, particularly Hatha or Anusara yoga, is beneficial to overall muscle flexibility. This specific pattern of poses, breathing, and relaxation is another great source of gentle, low-impact exercise. You may learn yoga from a videotape or through classes in your community. I recommend that you learn from a quiet, caring instructor in a small class setting.

Summary

This list is meant to inform you of Western and subtle energy therapies that may be appropriate in the support of your recovery. The decision about their effectiveness for your body is yours. Be proactive and self-responsible in your healing process. Participate, keep records, and journal your progress.

32

Nutrition and the Low Glycemic Diet

People either let things happen or they make things happen.

Dr. Amy Price, 2007

The fuel you offer your body has a tremendous impact on your recovery. Nutritional considerations foster a path toward physical health. You truly are what you eat, especially when the brain is sensitive to the fuel you offer.

This chapter discusses foods, vitamins, and herbs that enhance your body's ability to repair, heal and sustain itself. Any job is easier when the right tools are used.

You Are What You Eat

Certain foods will assist your healing process. Eat a "clean" diet. You already know the difference between brownies and lettuce. Eating clean means giving your body the best possible fuel. This is not a diet plan. This is what to eat and what not to eat. Pay attention. It's your new healthful, healing lifestyle plan.

Eat Clean

To me, "eating clean" means focusing on fresh foods, freshly prepared foods, unprocessed foods, and nutrition your body recognizes as food. Clean water is food. Coffee is not food. Whole-grain bread is food. Donuts are not food. You get the picture.

Eliminate the foods from your menu that are not genuine fuel for your body. Cut out white sugar, high-fructose corn syrup, all disguised sugar names, preserved or processed meat (hot dogs, lunch meat), anything fried, alcohol, chocolate, soda, and anything made with white flour. "Diet" foods are out, including anything sweetened with aspartame (Nutrasweet®) or sucralose (Splenda®). Rule out MSG (monosodium glutamate) when ordering Asian foods and any prepared food that relies on chemicals to enhance its taste. Rule out caffeine in any form: coffee, black tea, sweetened chocolate, soda pop. Rule out nitrates, nitrites, preservatives, or chemicals you don't recognize as safe. If you cannot pronounce it, do not eat it.

Rule out "fat-free" snacks, as the calorie count on these foods is disproportionately high. Rule out trans-fats, generally recognized as unhealthy. On the other hand, natural fats are very good for you. Vegetable fats like those found in avocados are genuine brain food, as are fish oils, olive oil and nuts. Cold water fish, such as wild salmon, are very good. Healthy fats are essential to building a healthy brain and a healthy body.[8]

Sweeteners such as stevia and xylitol work very well. In powdered and liquid form, they both have their place in your menu and palette. Different brands have slightly different tastes, so shop around. Generally I use stevia in tea and sprinkled on pancakes. I use xylitol for baking. (see "Brain Diet" chapter for recipes.)

The Low Glycemic Diet

Nutritional evidence is conclusively showing that, for most people, benefit abounds with following a "low glycemic" diet. I have long suspected that this way of organizing daily food intake is beneficial to the operation of the hypothalamus, the part of the brain that regulates, among other things, the perception of hunger. (This is the part of the brain that, because of its central location in the brain cavity, is generally involved in virtually all high-velocity brain-injury events, i.e., car crash, skull impact, trip and fall, baby-shaking, etc.)

Choose foods low in carbohydrates, high in fiber and fats, and lower in combustible calories than volume. This approach is known to moderate blood sugar, improve digestion, regulate and balance body weight and fat, regulate cholesterol levels to a degree, reduce overall stress, and greatly improve energy levels.

The next chapter will offer guidance onto this path. I have invented recipes that include all my husband's favorites (I won't try this diet unless it includes): pancakes, cookies, cake, waffles, and muffins. And chocolate. It's all low-carb and wonderful. You'll see.

Your Brain Will Crave Stimulants

In my years of private practice, there was always one telltale sign of brain-injured patients: their constant companion was a diet cola in hand.

Your body craves stimulants because your brain is constantly seeking an artificial kick-start. Your brain wants to work and craves activity. But the healing part of the brain needs you to be quiet so that the repairs can proceed in peace. Every can of soda you drink jars the system and slows down the repairs. Stimulants reduce the vitality of your immune system and over-rev your adrenal glands. (Don't get me started on sugar and artificial ingredients.)

Junk food is poison to your healing brain. Get it out of your body and out of your house. Eat clean.

Antioxidant Foods

Foods called "antioxidants" help to prevent the build-up of oxidation in your cells. (This is a very simplified explanation of a very complex process, but you can think of it this way. If you want to imagine the oxidation, think of the "rusty" appearance of an apple after you have bitten into it and left it sitting for a few hours.) Spirulina, blue-green algae, alfalfa tablets, soy foods, richly colored fruits and vegetables, and lecithin are good examples. Additive-free, carbonated waters may also be beneficial in moderation.

Broccoli is a good example of an antioxidant food. Whole grains that are high in vitamin E are beneficial as well. There are numerous books on this subject. Consult your neighborhood natural foods store for books, recipes, and ingredients.

Vitamins, Minerals, and Herbs

If broccoli is too much work or out of season, you can always obtain antioxidant formulas at a natural food store. In addition, infuse your system with zinc, the B complex, the C complex, Vitamin E, CoQ10, lecithin, gingko biloba, Gotu Kola herb, and ginseng herb. Also helpful are Bach Flower Remedies, especially Rescue Remedy. Homeopathic cell salts may be very helpful, as may be homeopathic nerve toners and nerve tonics. (Consult a homeopathic doctor.)

Anything known as a "brain food" will help. Warm milk or cooked turkey, both containing high levels of L-tryptophan, will assist in calming you. Non-stick coating for cooking pans is made of lecithin. Figs are calming and have a side benefit of reducing some forms of nasal congestion.

Food is positive fuel. Eat "brain food."

JANUARY 22, 1993

Nutritionally, I took lots of vitamins in addition to my already granola-head diet. Grains, green veggies (especially fresh spinach from my garden), fish, and lots of water were the mainstays. To that, I added a lot of B-complex, C-complex with bioflavinoids (strengthens blood vessel walls), vitamin E, vitamin A, zinc (repairs nerves), calcium-magnesium (builds bones and calms stress), lecithin (cleans blood, reduces cholesterol), niacin, and chromium picolinate (reduces cholesterol), psyllium seed husks (keep that colon squeaky clean!), and two very helpful extras: germanium (also sold as CoQ10) and proanthocyanidin (a.k.a. pycnogynol). Both are powerful antioxidants and brain-performance enhancers.

I also added some herbs, including valerian root, to repair the nervous system and allow for restful, uninterrupted sleep; Gotu Kola and ginkgo to clear my thinking and invigorate my brain; astragalus to boost the immune system; and ginger to stabilize and cleanse the blood and reduce visual dizziness and nausea.

I also noticed that chocolate and coffee were making their way into my diet. I had avoided caffeine all these years for the high allergic reaction I have consistently experienced, but now I discovered a craving for "coffee-flavored" things. Never drinking coffee outright, but coffee ice cream, mocha cake, espresso bean chocolates. I found the stimulation useful at times, in "medicinal doses." It's easy to overdo it, though.

I Confess

Yes, I consumed chocolate in medicinal doses. I also found that I became jittery, whiny, moody, and cranky if I abused it. This was not a fair trade to me, especially just before my period.

Luckily, with the advent of better chocolate products, it is actually possible to find dark chocolate with little or no sugar. Cocoa (cacao) is a very low carb food.

Once my metabolism leveled out, my brain was working better and I was feeling healthy again, I was able to add back in a bit of black tea, green tea, and some chocolate. All is not lost. With control and watchfulness, caffeinated foods may be added back in. At your own risk. Pay attention to the consequences.

Calories

You probably are less active than you were before your accident. You therefore need fewer calories for energy. Reduce the amounts of food you eat during this less-active time. Food is not your recreation.

Eat wisely. Chips and bon-bons are not going to offer you powerful fuel for healing. Drink lots of water. Juice and milk do not count. Drink 6 to 8 glasses of *water* per day, in addition to any milk, juice, or herbal tea. The exercise that will result from this regimen will keep you active.

Beware of late-night snacking. Eat your proteins early with dinner. The depressive, late-night carbo-munchies will not only add pounds of ugly fat to your hips, they will also disturb your sleep and burden your body when it needs to rest. Herbal tea is a better choice. And once you have mastered the low glycemic menu, your cravings will diminish or disappear.

Yeast Infections

When your brain function slows, your immune system can become depressed. This may lay you open to infections that seem to take forever to eradicate. Systemic yeast infections, sometimes known as Candida (a.k.a. *Candida albicans*), can grab a beachhead in your intestinal tract that not only will take forever to get rid of, but will mimic the symptoms of chronic fatigue syndrome. As if you weren't tired enough.

If you suspect Candida as the cause of your problem, naturopathic physicians can assist you in fighting this ailment with alternative medicines. The therapy generally includes a combination of food changes, vitamin therapy, herb therapy, and bodywork. It takes time, courage, and determination. It is hard enough to have a brain injury without giving up energy to an additional ailment.

I know, because Candida happened to me. I worked at getting rid of it for almost two years. The difference in energy levels was remarkable, and the effort was well worth it.

Be aware. Your immune system may become depressed. Infections and maladies that used to go away in a week may take longer to clear. Be vigilant about your health. Do not allow an ailment to drag on unattended. You can ill afford an additional chronic condition.

Visit your allopathic doctor (MD) for those maladies that fit the Western model. Antibiotics are a wonderful thing when you need them.

Most importantly, pay attention to your body. If you were unaware of the subtleties of your body before your accident, the injury may be compounding your ability to have active awareness now. Journaling is a good way to discover your level of awareness.

A variety of psychotherapy, exercise (like Tai chi, yoga), visualization methods (like EMDR, hypnosis, biofeedback), and meditation techniques may be valuable for building body awareness. Ask your support group therapy leader to spend some time discussing how to improve body awareness.

Summary

You are what you eat. Remain conscientious about the fuel you put in your body. Clean food just works better in the body. Come as close as you can to a clean diet. A little comfort food now and then is good for the soul, in medicinal doses. Eat well to get well.

33

The Healthy Brain Diet

I offer myself the gift of the Law of Attraction.

G. Denton, 2007

Low-Glycemic Menu Planning

Healthy body fuel sets the stage for a healthy brain, a vibrant body, and a creative and productive lifestyle.

These recipes and ideas were developed from my curiosity and creativity to satisfy my taste buds and metabolism. I was more concerned with the overall appropriateness of the ingredients than the "exact carb count" of a serving. Often I would watch the Food Channel and decide "I can do that low carb," then challenge myself to come up with a better recipe solution. What follows are ideas and recipes created from that inspiration. My research focused on various "Low Glycemic" and "Longevity" authors, who seem to agree that this menu path leads to a healthier, more vibrant, and longer, enjoyable life.

Mea Culpa: I am by tradition an eclectic scratch cook and create by eye, taste, and artistic bent. Some of these recipes are exactly measured, and others are free-form and up to you. Keep volume in mind. If something in the recipe sounds unbelievable, it might be. Keep your own counsel and create along with me! I hope you enjoy my culinary ventures.

The truth is, you will have to do some cooking, chopping, and stirring. It's worth it. You will be eating real, fresh food. Stay within the "low-glycemic" lists, recipes and menu plans the various authoritative books offer. (Yes, they will disagree on fine points. Choose from the spirit of the various opinions.) My goal is to eat about 60 grams of unprocessed carbohydrates per day, divided somewhat equally among the three meals of the day. I choose carb-free snacks.

You might need new kitchen tools. Sharp knives, several cutting boards, a simple egg poacher, blender, and food processor. Even with all this new gear and the amazing fresh ingredients, you will be surprised to discover that real food is less expensive than junk food. Really.

Rich, satisfying tastes are possible with the use of new seasonings, fresh herbs and spices, and new ingredients. This healthy journey will offer taste adventures that break you away from your old habits and offer you the gift of new, healthy, and delicious menus. As your taste buds shift to desiring higher-quality ingredients, your body will respond with increased energy, improved sleep cycles, and a healthful reserve of stamina. Your response to stressors may be more even, and your overall cognitive abilities can improve.

Get ready for your next adventure. Your body will thank you.

Take your glasses to the grocery store. You will be reading labels!

Recipe Sampler

Here is a tantalizing sampler by category of recipes and thoughts to get you started.

Appetizer

The appetizer, or starter, is a wonderful way to wake up your taste buds in preparation for a meal. Appetizers are generally meant to be a 3- to 5-bite experience, lively and direct.

Simple starters may include
   Celery sticks stuffed with almond butter
   Endive leaves stuffed with flavored cream cheese
   Quesadilla of chicken, avocado and Jarlsberg Lite cheese. Low-carb tortilla. Heat to melt cheese, fold, and serve, cut into wedges.

Shrimp Sushi Roll

Have fun making this great finger food!

1 cup cooked, chopped shrimp

1 cup ricotta cheese

Wasabi mustard for garnish

Black sesame seeds for garnish

1 cucumber, sliced long and skinny into strips (skin optional)

1 box sunflower sprouts, rinsed and patted dry

6 nori sheets (seaweed sheets)

Assemble by adding 1/6 of ingredients to each Nori sheet. Roll, moisten last 1/2" with water, roll and press together to seal. Slice, garnish with a sprinkle of black sesame seeds and Wasabi mustard on the side. Serve!

Soup

Soups, especially those with clear broth bases or those finished with cream, are filling, light, and delicious.

Simple soups may include

> Some Progresso soups are low carb, that is, under 20 grams per serving
>
> Clear broth with chopped veggies, heated and served
>
> Miso soup

Vietnamese Crab Soup

Sauté together the following:

1 shallot

6 asparagus spears, sliced

2 cups chopped Napa cabbage

1 carrot, sliced

2 tablespoons chopped cilantro

1 handful spinach leaves

2 teaspoons green chili, diced (canned or fresh—amount of heat to your discretion)

2 tablespoons olive oil

1 teaspoon sesame oil

Add in:

1 can crab meat

2 tablespoons fish sauce (soy sauce is ok)

Up to 4 cups chicken broth to cover all ingredients

Bring to a simmer.
Serve. Garnish with Thai basil leaves and a few shrimp (peeled-optional)
Serves 4.

Include a side of rye crackers with almond butter.
Option: For a more authentic look, scramble one egg and, just prior to serving, slowly drizzle it into the pot of simmering soup while stirring with a chopstick.

Salad

Fresh salads are the new centerpiece of your low-glycemic lifestyle. They come chilled, heated, chopped, shredded, sliced, and diced. Get out your knife, cutting board, salad spinner, and large bowl. Bring on the greens!

Simple salads may include
   Ready bagged salads, lettuces, romaine, spinach, Cole slaw, broccoli strips, carrot shreds, sprouts (Iceberg lettuce is the least nutritious "green")
   Classic tomato, cucumber, black olive, feta cheese, and olive oil
   Garnish with nuts, seeds, peas or garbanzo beans
   Mushrooms, jicama, avocado, diced apple, chopped grapefruit
   Turkey bacon, shredded cheese

Simple dressings may include
   Olive oil and balsamic vinegar
   Low-carb salad dressings (Beware the low-fat dressings. Read the label.)
   Lemon juice, lime juice, grapefruit juice, flax oil

Not salad
   Pasta, rice, potatoes, dry beans
   Gelatin desserts
   Iceberg lettuce

Hot Patty Pan Salad

Sauté with olive oil:
2 pounds patty pan squash, sliced: zucchini may be substituted
1/2 pound turkey bacon, chopped in 1" pieces
2 cups mushrooms, sliced

4 big handfuls spinach leaves

1 teaspoon Mrs. Dash seasoning

Place sautéed veggies in a serving bowl.

Add in:

1/2 cup feta cheese, crumbled

1 cup walnuts

2 tablespoons balsamic vinegar

Drizzle olive oil over the mixture

Dash of cayenne pepper or paprika

Toss and serve. Serves 4.

Entrée

Think of your entrée or central evening dish as the star of the menu. The leader of your dining enjoyment, the pacesetter of your lifestyle. Make it light, delicious, balanced, pleasing to the eye. Eat before 7 PM. Plan a walk after the meal.

Simple entrees may include

> Bison burger with low-carb bun or bread. (Great Harvest low-carb bread.)
> Chicken breast and steamed broccoli, salad
> Big salad with shrimp, chicken, or sliced steak
> Pizza made with low carb tortillas, or low carb pizza mix (Low-Carb Mix)
> Low-carb frozen entrée when you are on the go
> Turkey burger, chicken burger, lamb burger, ostrich burger!

Not dinner

> Fast food fare

Squid Steak Stir Fry

Sauté in olive oil:

1 large eggplant, cut into thin sticks (You may need to add in extra olive oil as this cooks up.)

Once the eggplant is tender, add in:

1/2 leek, cut into thin sticks

2 baby bok choy, cut into chunks

1 small green chili (or 2 tablespoons prepared diced green chilies from a can)

2 squid steaks, sliced into 1/4" strips

1 teaspoon Sambal chili sauce (optional)

1 tablespoon sesame oil

Once the squid strips are cooked, garnish with:

2 tablespoons cilantro, chopped

2 tablespoons soy sauce

Toss and serve. Serves 4.

OK, if squid steak is a challenge to find, this recipe works well with 1 pound of chicken strips, turkey strips, or pork strips.

Dessert

Of course you can have dessert! There are plenty of yummy treats out there that are good for you, delicious, and satisfying.

Simple dessert may include

    Fresh berries with coconut cream topping

    Homemade ice cream created with coconut milk and dark chocolate

    Cookies made with "Low-Carb Baking Mix"

    Dark chocolate, at least 70% or better cacao content

Healthful sweeteners

    Stevia, liquid or powder

    Xylitol crystals, used for baking and cooking

Not dessert

    Artificial sweeteners like Splenda®, Aspartame®, NutraSweet®, or products that contain them

Debi's Fool

Combine in a blender or food processor:

1 cup ricotta cheese

1 cup plain yogurt

1 teaspoon lemon zest

Juice of 1/2 lemon

1 tablespoon ground fresh ginger root

1/2 cup whipping cream

In a saucepan, combine:

Strawberries, blackberries, raspberries, and blueberries for a total of 36 ounces of fruit. Cook slightly and cool.

Add all ingredients to an ice cream maker. Follow directions for freezing. Serves 6.

Snacks

Almonds, cashews, walnuts, pecans, Macadamia nuts, Brazil nuts, and hazel-nuts (filberts) are all wonderful snacks. Focus on the fresh, unroasted, and unsalted products. Low in carbohydrates, high in healthful fats, a bag of nuts in your desk or day bag is a perfect snack treat. (Not peanuts. They are not a nut.)

Nut butters served with celery, carrots, apple slices, or other fresh dippers are also delicious, satisfying, and easy to manage.

Simple snacks may include
    Fresh berries
    Veggie sticks
    Small apple
    Nuts

Not snacks
    Junk food

Breakfast

A great day starts with a balanced breakfast, including protein. Your blood sugar gets its operating base from your breakfast choices. Focus on a simple, powerful and balanced meal.

Simple breakfast may include
    Poached egg on toast with butter
    Pancake topped with yogurt (Use the Low-Carb Baking Mix)
    Celery with almond butter or hazelnut butter
    Cucumber sticks with egg salad or tuna salad mix
    Salad with chopped boiled egg garnish

Not breakfast
    Toaster foods from processed ingredients
    Most "diet or breakfast drinks" and "breakfast bars"
    Bagels

Breakfast Basil

Sauté together in olive oil:
1 large Portobello mushroom, sliced

1 shallot, minced
4 stalks asparagus, chopped
1 handful spinach

Turn off heat, and add in:
1/4 cup feta cheese, crumbled
1 heaping tablespoon pesto

Toss, garnish with avocado slices, and serve. Serves 1.
(You may wish to top with a poached egg!)

Lunch

Hearty midday meals keep you nourished and alert. Fresh and crunchy ingredients rejuvenate.

Simple lunch may include

Salad with tuna, egg salad, shrimp, salmon garnish
Soup with veggie finger food
Yesterday's entrée leftovers
Salad bar

Confetti of Orange Roughy

Sauté together with olive oil:
1 cup celery, chopped
1/2 eggplant, stick sliced
1 cup red cabbage, chopped
1 medium zucchini, stick sliced
1 carrot, chopped
1 clove garlic

Add to top of sautéing vegetables:
1 pound orange Roughy fillets (sole, wild salmon, snapper, catfish OK)
Sprinkle vegetable seasoning on top of fish (Mrs. Dash, for instance)
Meanwhile, prepare a sauce.

In food processor combine:
1/2 cup cottage cheese
1/2 cup feta cheese, crumbled
2 teaspoons white truffle oil (optional)

Dash of cayenne pepper (paprika ok)

3-5 Kalamata olives, pitted (optional, and other olives will do)

Chill the sauce, and serve with entrée. Serves 4.

Dinner

Your third meal of the day works best when lighter. Plan to eat before 7 PM, to give your body the time to digest fully, relax, and prepare for evening rest.

Simple dinner may include

> Grilled meat and green salad
>
> Stew and chopped salad
>
> Turkey enchiladas and guacamole
>
> Entrée-size salad

Nothing says dinner like mashed potatoes. Here is your perfect choice for taste, texture, and carb-legal mashers.

Cauliflower Mashers

Steam until fully cooked:

1 cauliflower (florets of medium-size head)

In a separate pan, sauté with a bit of olive oil:

2 cloves garlic, minced

1 small shallot, minced

1 green onion, chopped (may substitute 2 tablespoons chopped chives)

Add together in a food processor (you may hand mash):

Steamed cauliflower

Sautéed items

1 tablespoon butter

1/3 cup Parmesan cheese, shredded

1 tablespoon olive oil

1-2 tablespoons sour cream (optional, and makes it really creamy)

2 teaspoons Mrs. Dash, or similar herbal seasoning mixture

Operate food processor until all ingredients are mixed and smooth.

Serve immediately. Makes 3-4 servings. (This recipe is not suited to leftovers.)

Great topped with a pan juice reduction. (To make a pan juice reduction, remove your cooked meat, deglaze with red wine. When the wine has cooked down sufficiently, finish with a small pat of butter. Stir and pour over your cauliflower mashers.) So yummy.

Beverages

The carbs really add up with juice, soft drinks, fancy coffee, "umbrella drinks," and cocktails. Remember beverage content as you observe your daily food intake.

Artificial creamers, artificial sweeteners, premixed adult beverages, and flavored coffees carry carbohydrates. Some fancy water products are loaded with carbs and artificial ingredients.

Simple beverages may include

    Black coffee

    Green tea, black tea, and herbal tea

    Iced coffee or tea you make yourself

    Diluted juice drinks, with less than 25% juice

    Water: 8 glasses a day

    Wine Spritzer: 1/4 wine, 3/4 Club soda

Quick Breads

The low-carb baking mix was my first low-carb recipe. The main goal was to create a low-carb path towards pancakes, cookies, breads, muffins, cakes, and crackers that met the low-carb/unprocessed-carb criteria and the family taste-bud requirement.

Low-Carb Baking Mix

In a large mixing bowl combine:

1 cup wheat germ

1 cup oat flour

1 cup oat bran

1 cup flax meal

1 cup almond flour

1 teaspoon salt

4 teaspoons baking powder

4 tablespoons egg white powder

2 teaspoons freshly ground nutmeg

Combine all dry ingredients and store refrigerated in an airtight container.

Use these ingredients to make other things: for pancakes, for each cup of mix, add in 1 egg and 2 tablespoons olive oil. Mix, and add in enough water or milk to make a smooth pancake mix. Set it aside for 10 minutes, as it will absorb the liquid. Now add in enough more liquid to thin the batter to your use. Pancakes, waffles, muffins.

Vitamin Strategy

Vitamins, minerals, herbal formulas, and supplements may be a part of your daily regimen. Consider spreading the doses out rather than taking everything all at once. Your body will have a better chance of assimilating the nutrients when taken at different times.

Think about taking your supplements with breakfast and lunch. Many supplements are stimulating and not suited to evening consumption. Listen to your body and do what works best, or with a practitioners guidance.

Essential fatty acids, the omega oils, are vital to brain health. When taking cod liver oil, I found that chewing a few black olives quickly thereafter cleared the oil taste from my palette. When taking encapsulated oils, I kept shopping until I found a brand of omega 3s that sat well with my tummy.

Ingredient Resources

Where will you find all these new, low-carbohydrate, unprocessed foods? In some cases, these items are in abundance in your local grocery store. The produce aisle will become your new best friend!

Other items are found in natural food stores, in the natural food aisle of your grocery store, a local Asian market, a local Mexican market, and of course on-line. There are natural food cooperative buying clubs available on-line.

In many states, there are cooperative vegetable farms that offer harvest shares. You can usually find out about these at a local farmer's market. The produce is grown locally and organically and picked fresh. You can search on-line for a "CSA" (Community Supported Agriculture) to find farms in your area.

34

Trauma, Recovery, and the Newly Fragile You

Just as we are each the sum total of our lifetime experiences, so too are we the sum total of our bumps, scrapes, and traumatic events. The difference is, with life experience, you can make good cocktail party conversation. With bumps and trauma, the record is imbedded in the nervous system and accumulates with the intensity of each additional event. The net effect is cumulative sensitivity to all subsequent traumatic events.

Lifetime Cumulative Effects

This phenomenon is of particular importance as you move forward in life. Between your head injury, that fall on the ice last winter, the anesthesia from a recent surgery, trips to the dentist, and whacking your head in the garage last spring, it adds up significantly. Your body may respond more slowly to recovery from each ensuing incident. The gravity of all subsequent insults builds upon previous injury. You develop a fragile overall response. You become an active collection of physical and emotional trauma.

If you are in litigation proceedings, it is imperative that your attorney understands this phenomenon, not only for explaining the effects of your life in relation to the issue at court, but for clearly demonstrating the consequences for you moving forward in life (and the necessary support projected for your future.)

Mild Traumatic Brain Injury Versus Posttraumatic Stress Disorder

Along with mild traumatic brain injury, which is essentially a physical injury, it is possible to develop posttraumatic stress disorder, which is basically an emotional response to trauma. When the acquisition of the brain injury includes a violent scene (horrific car crash, domestic abuse, roadside explosion), that visual or emotional image lodges with the individual. Played over and over in the mind and recorded in body memory, posttraumatic stress disorder can become a significant piece of the brain-injury recovery scenario.

I suspect that over time, as we observe military service members returning from war experiences, the incidence of mild traumatic brain injury with posttraumatic stress disorder will be remarkable. My hope is that our service members will be adequately diagnosed and treated for all their wounds.

Summary

Now more than ever, you are the sum total of your experiences and parts. Unlike the experiences of the general population, however, your traumatic experiences will weigh more heavily upon your lifetime record. Live with awareness and peaceful observation, and seek therapeutic relief from your bumps and crunches. You may require more trips to the chiropractor, massage therapist, or cranial-sacral practitioner. OK, then go. Routine maintenance is crucial to addressing those potholes and keeping you as active as possible.

Treat yourself gently, with support and therapy as indicated. You'll just need it a little more often.

35

Dental Strategies

Dental health is essential to overall physical health. It's easy to postpone regular dental visits with the multitude of therapies and lifestyle stresses with which a brain-injured person must deal. This is precisely why the dentist is a valuable member of your recovery team!

Overall stress puts pressure on the general state of your oral hygiene. Because body chemistry may have shifted, gum and tooth health may be affected. Dental-hygiene visits every 6 months are essential to maintain and support your overall health. This strategy screens for tooth health, cavities, gum and tongue health, and possible grinding from stress or TMJ (jaw-joint pain).

Pick the Right Dentist

Paramount to your positive dental experience is choosing a dentist sensitive to brain-injury issues. You might be making unique requests, need to take breaks during your session, request extra pillows, or have various noise or lighting considerations. Review these special needs. Change dentists if cooperation is not forthcoming.

Previsit Preparation

Consider making your appointment in the morning. This gives you the whole day to actively recover from the effects of the visit. Make sure to have a breakfast with protein ingredients. Drink plenty of water. Take at least 1000 mg of vitamin C before the appointment.

What to Take to the Visit

Be prepared for your visit. Wear comfortable clothes. In the summer, I take a beach towel and spread it on the leather chair for comfort. Take your sunglasses in with you, and a hat with a visor. These items really help shade you from the overhead exam light as well as the general lighting in the room (which is usually fluorescent). You may also bring ear plugs to shield your ears from drill noise. These items reduce your exposure to overstimulating environmental input.

Pillow Strategies in the Chair

Reclining in a dental chair for an hour or more can easily stress your neck and back, and has a way of triggering TMJ pain . Request a neck pillow and a knee pillow and feel free to fuss with them until they are comfortable and right for you. Ask for a break when you need one and also readjust the pillows when necessary. When I know I'm in for a two-hour session at the dentist, I make a chiropractic or a massage appointment for the next day.

Dental Anesthesias

Dentists have a wide range of choices for anesthesia. The "Novocaine-style" injections into the oral cavity actually have varying ingredients. One includes epinephrine (also called adrenaline), which triggers a response in some people. This choice may be very agitating to a brain-injured person, whose adrenal function may already be stretched to the limit! Avoid this anesthetic agent in the future if you experience an agitated response. Have your choice recorded in your dental chart.

Some dentists offer nitrous oxide gas, which can relax you. This anesthetic, which you breathe in, may make your brain "fuzzy" for the rest of the day. If you choose this type of anesthesia, take note of the aftereffects during the rest of your day. Have your choice recorded in your dental chart.

After the Dental Visit

To soften the effects of a dental visit, drink lots of water, take another 1000 mg vitamin C, and consider taking Rescue Remedy. A protein drink, miso soup, or clear broth will give you support to quickly move any drugs that you received during the dental procedure out of your system.

The Mouth Guard

Many brain-injured people develop a jaw clenching or night teeth grinding behavior that is damaging over time to your teeth and jaw joints. Left unaddressed this behavior leads to damaged cracked teeth, possible root canal work, intractable TMJ, sinus involvement, constant headaches, neck pain, and nervous exhaustion.

A simple tool to relieve stress from this painful and destructive cycle is the addition of a mouth guard or mouth splint. Worn mostly at night, yet also worn during the daytime if that helps, it is a simple plastic device that fits over either the lower or upper teeth. It's clear and has the same general feel of an orthodontic retainer. Its main purpose is to protect your teeth and to keep your jaw from clamping down all the way in its range of motion.

I highly recommend the lower-jaw splint. Most dentists are used to making the upper-jaw splint and may not initially cooperate with your request for a lower-jaw splint. In fact, the lower-jaw splint works best for most brain-injured people. It protects your teeth without engaging the structure of the skull or the subtle movements of the scalp. It is less invasive. Your cranial-sacral therapist will notice the supportive difference.

Some dental plans support the cost of this device.

Summary

Healthy teeth are vital to overall vitality. See your dentist regularly. Floss daily. Be prepared with comfort items that support your visit to the dentist.

36

Fatigue Syndromes

You are now living a sensitive, gently alert, and softly vigilant life. Paramount to long-term healthy and vibrant patterns is an awareness of your general energy level and an active noticing of dips, swings, and gullies of fatigue.

It's one thing to be tired occasionally, for a day or a few days. However, when fatigue sets in for a long stretch, it is appropriate to take notice and take action. Of course, there are different sorts of fatigue caused by differing factors.

Brain-Injury Fatigue

With a brain injury comes physiologic suppression. Your body wants you to be still while it sends healing energy to the brain. This is a normal, appropriate response to the situation for your body to safeguard you during healing. You may feel fuzzy or lethargic, but, as your injury resolves, this situational fatigue should lift over time.

Depression-based Fatigue

When situational fatigue has difficulty resolving—and continues beyond reasonable parameters (based on the grade of brain injury you sustained) of positive resolution—initial fatigue can develop into a more complex issue, including clinical depression. Helped by various tests (including 24-hour saliva and urine tests to discover your brain chemistry levels), your psychiatrist can choose an antidepressant appropriate for your case.

Antidepressants are made of different ingredients to address different body-chemistry needs. Be confident that the medication you choose with your doctor is the correct medicine for your brain and body situation. Do not be content with a "desperation" pill prescribed by a frustrated family practitioner eager to "try something." Keep working at it until the doctor can tell you exactly why the prescription is the best attempt.

Chronic Fatigue Syndrome

Chronic fatigue is a more long-term, cascading complex of multiple issues. The result is long-term fatigue and a mixed puzzle of symptoms, complaints, and medical issues. Causing constant fragility and exhaustion, and the inability to sustain cognitive function for more than brief periods of time, chronic fatigue feels like a dark hole.

Extrication from chronic fatigue takes a team of cooperating practitioners and your resolve to stay committed to the process, however long it takes and whatever the rules might be for you. Choose a team that includes alternative medical practitioners, Western medical practitioners, a nutritionist who understands the benefits of the low-glycemic regime for brain injury, exercise, and psychotherapy for positive visualization. Select the best from among the available therapists in your area.

Adrenal Fatigue Syndrome

Adrenal fatigue is a more recently identified cascading complex of multiple issues centering on the exhaustion of the adrenal system. Healthy adrenal glands secrete adrenaline when your body experiences a "fight or flight" situation. Brain injury can cause this normal response to trigger so frequently the adrenal glands eventually fire constantly. As you live on a steady diet of adrenaline, of course it exhausts the overworked glands and you.

You may feel completely exhausted yet agitated, jumpy, raw, and irritated all the time. It wears you out just being you. There are numerous books available addressing this syndrome. Adrenal fatigue is considered "sub-clinical" by Western medicine. Diagnosis usually includes a 24-hour saliva test.

Long-term remedy includes supplements, diet and lifestyle habit shifts, exercise, and rest. Because it took time for your body to get into this condition, it will take time to rehabilitate. Be patient and constant. Follow the suggestions with the guidance of your support system.

I acquired adrenal fatigue syndrome and followed the combined advice in three publications. I selected the suggestions that sounded true for me. With 6 months of faithful adherence, I began to get my energy and my lifestyle back.

Infection-based Fatigue

Low-grade infections can slowly and silently debilitate energy and stamina. Yeast infections, intestinal Candida, even an infected tooth can slowly grind away at energy. It is helpful to screen for these issues while examining for other fatigue issues. Sub-clinical infection may not stand out in a field of symptoms, but it can be a mystery puzzle piece.

Realizations for Long-Term TBI Lifestyles

As your life progresses forward and you learn to live a positive and productive life with a brain injury, know that observation and quiet, alert overview supports your general health and future plans. The New You will have a few vulnerabilities that, when supported and watched, remain healthy members of your body. If fatigue sets in, know that resolution is possible.

Summary

Should you be susceptible to fatigue in its various forms, know that the path forward exists. Your fragile constitution can respond to support and lifestyle choices. There are solutions to these complex issues. Resolution takes time. Ultimately, your lifestyle will improve, energy can return, and your overall body awareness and alertness will serve you well in the years to come.

Part VI

THE EMOTIONAL BODY

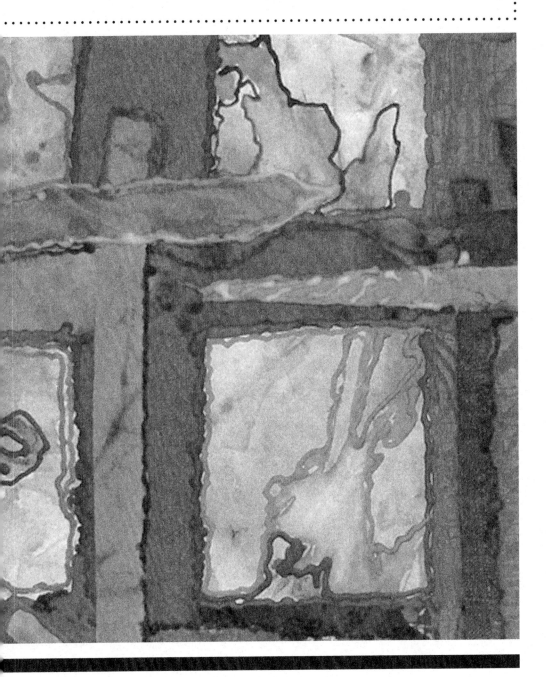

37

Emotions and Denial

A roller coaster of emotional experience may accompany the effects of depression during your recovery. Emotional factors are widespread and encompass the breadth of your environment. Issues of control, restlessness, vulnerability, sadness, helplessness, hopelessness, embarrassment, agitation, and denial can all be facets of this roller-coaster ride. It's as if, in the process of properly putting all the parts back together, some parts lay chilled on the floor far too long.

Your emotions are extremely important. They can be fueled by an overactive imagination, which exhausts and potentially frightens. This chapter will explore the feelings that accompany your brain injury. It will also give you some ideas about how to cope with and utilize your emotions to achieve a positive outcome.

The Laundry List of Emotions

You will be familiar with most of these emotions because you have experienced them in your life before. Some emotions will be ones that you may not have fully experienced before. There may also be emotional intensities greater than your general expectancy. Brain injury will magnify the emotions. You are powerless to modulate these emotions. You are tired.

Fatigue also magnifies the emotional experience, sometimes taking emotional response to a realm that feels out of control. This fatigue is enhanced because of the unpredictability you experience on a daily basis. You are too tired to filter and discern.

Cultural Shame

Long-term illness is denied in American culture. Our cultural myth focuses upon the young, strong, healthy, and bootstrap-energized hero, armed with the Constitution and free to explore the far horizons. In America, if you are sick, you had better darn well look sick. In America, there is a two-week limit on sore throats and flu and an eight-week limit for the use of crutches. Beyond that, and you are pretty much faking. Without tubes in your nose or a wheelchair to sit in, you are not sick.

Consequently, our culture has no way to gauge long-term illness that is not readily apparent. You, personally, have no way to gauge your long-term illness and no measure or guide for how to fit in. There is no ready example for conduct. There is only shame. Embarrassment is added to the list of emotions with which we must cope.

Embarrassment

Externally you look "fine," even "normal." Look in the mirror and see that you even look fine to yourself. Who can tell that you are ill or differently abled? So, in addition to being embarrassed by your newly discovered emotional aspects, you now experience anger over having to feel embarrassed by something that isn't even your fault. Add onto that the anxiety over the embarrassment, then finally the worry of it all, and you have a giant jumble of emotions stemming solely from a lack of cultural support for what you are going through.

This is not very good news, but hopefully it will explain the environment you are likely to encounter. Our culture fails to recognize our dilemma and our pain. We must be crazy. There is no other cultural explanation. Clearly, we are making this all up.

Irritability

Your emotional "fuse" will shorten considerably with brain injury. Disorientation, coupled with fatigue, will shorten anyone's patience. With continuous pressure, your fuse will remain short for a considerable length of time. Being perceived as crazy doesn't help.

The more you learn about your energy resources, the more able you will be to regulate and modulate your behavior. (See the chapter "Stamina, Fatigue, and Energy.")

Agitation

Before my injury, I never thought of myself as feeling like the inside of an old fashioned washing machine. They don't call it the agitator for nothing. Sometimes the combination of stress and pressure can result in that feeling of being wound up, releasing, and winding up again for another round. Agitation has no escape. I did notice, however, that when I acknowledged that I was agitated, the feeling reduced a bit. Sometimes, the relief of identifying the feeling induces calm. Try it.

Identify the Feeling

Identification is accomplished by yourself or with the help of a support person. Answer the question: What am I feeling now? It may help, in the beginning, to write down any and all feelings the moment you experience them. The more practice you have understanding your feelings, the better you will become at pinpointing and describing them. You may or may not be able to do anything about the feelings, but identification induces a sense of calm and control. Naming the feelings empowers the experience.

Remember, if your list of feelings is long or enmeshed, include *feeling overwhelmed* on the list.

Restlessness

That fidgety feeling may creep into your life. A sense of urgency or of impending action or doom may occur, but you have no idea why. This feeling may lapse over into nighttime and keep you from sleeping. Sleeping aids generally cannot touch restlessness. Calming music or rhythmic breathing help.

Anger

There are generally two kinds of anger associated with brain injury.

(1) The first kind of anger is most obvious. Your life, your mind, your emotions, your work, and your personal universe have been altered. Simply

stated, this is not fair. You have a perfect right to be angry. Life is suddenly a puzzling struggle in a dark tunnel. Definitely something to be legitimately angry about.

(2) The second sort of anger is more generic and appears less logical. It is the anger that we could regulate with sophisticated social skills, but that now comes bursting out beyond our control. It is unattractive, embarrassing, unpredictable, inappropriate, and brutally honest. Simply stated, this is not fair either.

If anger was never an acceptable behavior in your life, your challenge in dealing with it now will be harder work and probably terrifying. If anger was an acceptable emotion in your house, I am sure we will find something else on this list to keep you busy.

If anger is a serious issue for you, discuss it with your psychotherapist. It is no coincidence that there is a therapy category called "anger work". Be sure to remind your psychotherapist that you have limited energy means due to your brain injury. Traditional focused "anger work" may not be appropriate or well timed. (See the chapter "Anger and Forgiveness.")

Posttraumatic Stress Disorder

Within your injury diagnosis, you may be carrying what is called an "overlay" of stress from your accident. Posttraumatic stress disorder hangs like a cloud over recovery. It is a condition characterized by recurring, unresolved psychological responses to overwhelming experiences like an accident or war service. The individual is in a continual repetitive loop of events or flashbacks and the subsequent trauma, exhaustion, and debilitating anguish that result. Left untreated, permanent emotional disability results.

NOVEMBER 17, 1992

Sometimes it feels like a hand grenade was thrown into my life and the shrapnel keeps showing up in the cookies. Back to the dentist with another cracked tooth.

As if the map is changed so often, I have decided to just camp here until the spinning stops. Do not ask me to go for a walk. The tent may have moved in the meantime.

There may be layers of trauma that you cannot see or feel. Those layers will eventually reveal themselves. Your best defense is to know that the layers will work themselves out. Welcome the layers. They indicate the path to recovery.

Sadness

Some days you may just feel sad. That is OK. Resist the temptation to explain or justify it. It is normal to feel sad. It happens. It will go away. Phony attempts to cheer you up will not work.

Vulnerability

I used to get this "tiny little bird" feeling. I felt fragile, unprotected, undefended, exposed, and an easy target. That cold, wet, hungry, helpless feeling would wash over me, and I would shut down. Many times I would not leave the house except to fetch the mail. For some reason, there was a safety zone on the path to the mailbox.

The truth is, vulnerability is a reasonable response to brain injury. The brain is not as alert as usual. Protective vigilance is reduced. Thinking is slowed and vulnerability is an issue. Remember that this feeling of fragility is exaggerated by your mental state. Yes, you are a bit more vulnerable, but not nearly as much as you presently perceive.

Remember: "I am safe." "I have a support system." "This is a safe place."

Fear of Death

Overactive imagination and depression, though quite different from one another, can contribute to a feeling of dread and impending death. While both are different from premonitions and paranormal experiences, neither is to be ignored. Doom is a part of the depression landscape and must be clinically addressed. Seek medical help immediately if your sense of hope is lost, or you have unresolved feelings of dread or impending doom.

Mood Swings

When you experience large gulfs between happiness and despair within a short period of time, you are experiencing mood swings. Crying easily or crying often are also signals of mood swing. Generally, moods are swinging when states of being are radically shifted from positive to negative (or vice versa). This generally feels like a roller coaster ride and may be accompanied by "poor me" times, crying, hysterical laughing, a short-fuse remark, or other emotional displays that are out of control or inappropriate.

Mood swings bring up memories of being ambushed or being taken by surprise. Sometimes it feels as if you are possessed and another being is acting out through you. At times, it can even feel as though you are watching the event unfold before you and you are helpless to stop it. Yes, it can feel weird. I swear I have an evil twin.

After two years of mood swings, I began to be able to predict their arrival. In a way similar to epileptics who can sense the onset of a seizure, I began to sense when a mood swing was approaching. I would call my spouse to hold me. With his support, and by talking the feelings through, I am now able to get through these events with a little more dignity and control. Most of the time, anyway. (See "Limbic Rage.")

Hypochondria, Menopause, and Other Drama

Along with all the other hypersensitivity of this experience, you may notice that you think you are contracting all sorts of additional illnesses. My body clock was so messed up, I thought I was entering menopause. I did check it out, first with my mother to see what the going age was in our family. Then, I went to the gynecologist for a check-up. She suggested that the accident may have rerouted my hormones temporarily. This can happen.

After fixating on breast cancer for a month, I went for a mammogram. That set my mind to rest also.

Even getting a cold or the flu can feel much bigger than it ever felt before. Checking with a family member first, someone who knows what you act like when you get sick, is a good place to start. If you really are sick, then certainly go to the doctor. Simply know that the perception of common illness may be exaggerated by your sensory system.

Overactive Imagination

Your mind is very powerful. In fact it can be so powerful that stories, plots, and worst-case scenarios that would normally be filtered out now come popping to the surface. And you believe them to be true!

You may even tell these wild stories to others, believing them to be true. You may also embellish real stories so that they have a more interesting ending. This tends to occur because your judgment and discernment are under funded and your imagination is literally running wild.

Jumpiness

Generic fear surfaces most often when you are alone, reacting to the things that go bump in the night. You may feel a presence in the house or a feeling of being observed. It may also manifest itself when you are around people but not aware of their proximity. Being startled easily is an example. Our sense of proximity or our location relative to others is miscalculated. This produces a sense of jumpiness or positional insecurity. It feels unsafe.

It happens because our senses are operating poorly. Jumpiness will subside as the senses heal. That feeling of general safety and emotional stability will gradually return.

Emotional Liability

When life seems like one long crying jag, feeling like an emotional liability can occur. You are not any fun to be around. Everyone has to tippy-toe around the house. Life is a drag and you are the cause. The whole mess is a marathon of exhaustion. Pressure comes from everywhere, and overwhelm nips at its heels.

Your friends likely have unconsciously given you a certain amount of time to get well, and you have not lived up to those expectations. You do look fine. But you are not the same person, and you are not yet able to perform to expectations. Feeling overwhelmed is easy.

Resist the belief that you are a liability. You are doing the best you can, and it happens to fit only your timetable. Your timetable is enough in the face of this unpredictable experience. Rest and heal, andremind your friends that you are still in the healing process. Applying yourself daily.

Denial

There are two main parts to denial.

(1) The first denial is about whether or not you had a brain injury. Deny it all you want. The longer you deny it, the longer you postpone recovery.

(2) The second part of denial focuses on acknowledging the new you. Acceptance of your evolving new self is vital to recovery. Challenges occur daily, especially if the new you is behaving in an unfamiliar, embarrassing, or uninhibited manner. The new you may not always be pretty or recognizable.

The challenge of accepting your new self centers around grieving the loss of the parts that may not return **and** welcoming the new parts. Ultimately your self-esteem will rest on how much you love the new you.

Certainly there is regret over the loss of parts you liked about yourself. You may also have lucked out and lost parts that you will not miss. Notice the gift of what you have gained in the process. For instance, I became less critical of myself and others. (That is a nice thing to lose.) I became more artistic. (That is a nice aspect to gain.) A good trade, all in all.

Grief and loss are topics to discuss with your psychotherapist. Developing self-esteem around the new you is a valuable topic. If you are in group therapy, self-esteem for the new you is a perfect topic to discuss. Feedback from others will give you support for the formation of a fresh personal image.

Silent Suffering

Mild brain injury is a fairly invisible illness. It may even feel anonymous, the unseen and forgettable malady. You could be struggling in silence a good deal of the time. Others will not readily know you are struggling. Brain injury is simply not that obvious to others, no matter how omnipresent, insidious, and all-encompassing it is in your life.

However, you are not being persecuted. Recovery is about telling the truth, asking for support, and moving on as best you can. If you are invisible to others, positive enrollment of their support is in order. Ask for help, ask for accommodation, and resist asking for sympathy. It uses up vital energy that could be more productively allocated. (See the chapter "Support Systems.")

Loving Your (New) Self

Slowly and steadily you will discover your (new) self. Your (new) self is the new person emerging during your healing process. Welcome the new you every chance you get. "I joyously welcome my new self."

I love to visit Utah in the springtime and sit in the desert. It is so amazingly quiet, you can almost hear the stars come out at night. I began to uncover my new self there, as shared through this journal entry.

APRIL, 10, 1992

The only true danger in the desert, aside from bumble bees the size of a Buick, or if you happen to be Frank the Plastic Flamingo and lose the battle of the gusty wind, winding up with one leg, a splinted neck, and wing reconstruction surgery, is what you may hear from inside your own head: whatever you suppress with your everyday activity, noise and chatter that keeps you from your ugly and frightening self-truths. Truths that we all have. Truths that are just that. Just truths. Thoughts. Demons in the air. Feelings about which rewritten history can heal whole chapters in a deep second. Truth that does not keep others from loving you, but only you from loving yourself. Truths that need no longer be your truth. Truths that only need be your history, not your destiny.

Take a moment in the desert for deep personal ecology. Discover the timeless blessing of clean peace, soul-cleansing quiet, blissful personal regard, private unconditional love. And notice that it is your new reality.

Panic Attacks

The sudden onset of a panic attack can be frightening, especially if you have neither seen nor experienced one before. A panic attack takes many forms. Tight breathing, the feel of a weight on the chest, the "fight or flight" response, complete vulnerability, and an "out of control" feeling are among the aspects of panic attack.

A few signs of panic attack are bizarre or "this is not me" behaviors such as assuming the fetal position, hiding in a closet or under a bed, an inability to verbally respond, being suspended in a nonverbal state, exhibiting nonadult behaviors, talking too loudly, uncontrolled sobbing, and hyperventilating.

A panic attack is triggered by your emotions. It can strike at any time and respects no circumstance. Ordinarily a panic attack demands your full attention. Resisting creates a stronger rebounding experience. Know that you will be OK when it is over. Place no judgment on the experience. Ask for support. Inform your healthcare team. Rest and recover. A panic attack uses a tremendous amount of energy, of which you have precious little. This too shall pass.

Unconscious Incompetence

The tremendous effort of living life with a brain injury runs headlong into the unconscious world of people we will meet along the way. These folks lope along, operating at an average level of competency. Their poor effort squanders our limited time, resources, energy, and patience.

When I am trying so intently to get it right, using every ounce of strength to move through the day, I have been known to "lose it" when confronted by below-average performance or lackluster service. With full effort engaged to plod through the moment, I am puzzled by less than full effort in others. I pay a higher price for the services rendered than the service providers in the performance of their task. My consequences are expensive.

Over the years, I have struggled with my response to this situation. The answers are not easy. The strategy is to consume minimal energy under the circumstances.

Summary

Your (new) self will emerge as you heal. It will have new aspects, and there will be missing aspects from your former self. Explore, discover and accept this new person. This is the path of your life now. It is your new reality. Embrace it and move powerfully forward.

38

Depression

The human body will do everything in its power to heal itself. Mild, temporary, emotional distress is a normal human occurrence. Hormone changes, loss of a loved one, job change, or nutrition deficiency can bring about the "blues." This happens to us all at one time or another. It is generally referred to as *"situational"* depression.

On the other hand, depression from brain injury is entirely different. It may last for months or years. Because you may have never before experienced long-term depression, this factor alone can be a tremendous challenge in your recovery process. The illness of depression leads to a downward emotional spiral that is potentially very dangerous and must be professionally addressed and treated.

This chapter discusses the many forms that depression can take and how to understand, recognize, and cope with them for as long as they are needed in the healing process.

Depression

There is a tremendous difference between being bummed out that your plant died or your picnic was rained out and the devastating effects of true depression. Depression lasts, and, in the event of brain injury, depression is debilitating. The injury to your brain upsets the natural balance of the brain's neurotransmitters, which modulate your mood. This imbalance creates what is known as *"organic"* depression, the hallmark of which is a loss of a sense of hope.

Secondly, if you are further stressed by a life event such as a major change in your level of functioning, you may develop a "***reactive***" depression. If it persists long enough, a reactive depression can also develop into a biochemical imbalance that will deepen your current depression.

This journal entry encapsulates it for me.

JANUARY 31, 1992

> There were times of profound stress. Times of frozen activity. Moments, hours, and days halted by a thought that would not connect. By a body too tired, too confused, or too exhausted and confused to continue.

If depression figures heavily in your experience and you seek medication, please remember this: depression is often misinterpreted in brain injury. Depression symptoms mimic so many different diagnostic choices. The complication of brain injury as the source of the problem is often overlooked, discounted, or ignored. Make sure your doctor understands that your depression is likely a result of brain injury rather than emotional or environmental sources. Also, be very sure that you understand and accept that you may experience some side effects from your prescribed medication. Sometimes it takes several trials of different medication to find the ones that work well with *your* neurochemistry. Be sure to report unpleasant side effects to your doctor immediately. I recommend seeking a psychiatrist with experience in brain-injury treatment.

JOURNAL ENTRY MAY 12, 2007

> So far, three doctors have offered me antidepressants. I'm spiraling badly and a legion of appointments has not solved the riddle. But a small voice inside tells me not to accept the prescription until someone can tell me exactly why the medication is appropriate.
>
> Finally, armed with blood tests and saliva tests showing levels of brain chemicals really high or really low and definitely out of whack, a psychiatrist familiar with brain injury puts the puzzle pieces together. She can tell me exactly why the selected antidepressant is appropriate. OK. Now I'll take it.

The same is true for psychotherapy. Make sure your practitioner understands that your depression is probably a biochemical response to brain injury. Standard depression therapies may not be appropriate, too exhausting, or cognitively overwhelming. Most appropriate are action-oriented and problem-solving therapy approaches designed to explore self-esteem issues, coping strategies, support-system building, compensation skills, and relationship development.

Ideations

An overstimulated and overactive imagination combined with low self-esteem and depression can create a worry cycle, or exhausting "what if" ideation cycle. If, in addition, you experience a biochemical imbalance, you may get caught in a process called rumination, or more emphatically, perseveration. This occurs when one's thinking unproductively goes over and over the same issues with no clear resolution or end.

JUNE 6, 1992

> With recovery has come not only the visible depression and upset of life alterations and low mental energy, but occasional, random visualizations/thoughts/inklings that creep into my reasonable train of thought and hold violent/disrupting/self-esteem—eroding/self-doubting ideas. Almost bushwhacked by the feelings. Sometimes sucked right into the thought mode. Sometimes believing it. I am not enough. Things are not going to work out. I am not lovable. He will leave me for sure. I cannot think or remember. I cannot protect myself. I won't get well.
>
> These are the silent assassins in my brain. They slip in and out from among the shadows of my mind, throwing in a banana peel or a handful of buckshot. Reminds me of a highway sign in southern Idaho that warns: *Occasional Blinding Dust Storms.* Almost an off-hand remark, except for the kicker.

Ideation, like vision issues, are singular facets of depression, yet important enough to devote an entire chapter to. (See the chapters "But What If...... Ideations" and "Vision.")

"On the Edge of Screaming Tears"

I found this phrase written on a slip of green paper that was tucked into my notebook. It was definitely my handwriting. I have been to that point frequently during the depression. It does help to scream sometimes. Usually, a big fluffy pillow is a good place to deposit the outburst. I tried it while driving but found that a poor idea. Not only was it cognitive overload (driving and screaming), I parched my throat and could not talk for a day afterward. Letting out this sort of anguish is best done in privacy. There are more tissues handy: a safe place to cry, sob, and gently gain comfort and composure.

Crying may be a new or rediscovered experience for many of you. Your best bet is to accept it into your life for the time being. It provides a beneficial avenue for release, frustration, and anger. It may not be how you picture yourself, and you may have held judgments against criers. It is a useful and fruitful response to your present, temporary condition. Tears cleanse and release.

However, you may wish to share your emotional pain with someone you trust. A compassionate psychologist who can offer genuine support and reliable feedback would be ideal. You can offer yourself the experience and opportunity of knowing that you are acceptable as a human being, even in this most unglamorous state. Sometimes you will not be able to hold back your tears, and sometimes tears will come for seemingly no reason. Keep your tissues handy, and use this reaction as useful feedback that your brain is overloaded. You need to take a serious break and honor your healing process.

If you find that your partner discounts your information when you are crying, remember: ***his or her reaction is not about you***. What you have to say is valid. Your delivery system is doing its best at the moment.

Mulling and Worrying

The constant thread that runs through the mind of the depressed person is the vulnerability, lack of control, and loss of hope in one's life. I found myself evolving into a worry wart. You may find yourself in the whirlpool of your mind, just as I did.

APRIL 27, 1993

My mind mulls. Everything. Especially bad things. Like breast cancer. And a list of social ills. And violent scenes in movies and on the news. For days. Weeks.

Breast cancer is frightening. No one in my family on either side for two generations has had it. I am very low profile to get it, as far as the brochures say. I self-exam, get mammograms, and have Pap exams regularly. Do not smoke or take birth control pills. But, I have never had a baby. That is where the odds change.

This turns in my mind incessantly. Then another lobe chimes in, "You get what you fear," so then I wonder if I am giving it to myself through worry. How can I shut off the worry?

Then there are the movie flashbacks. I avoid obviously violent films, but even comedy slips in a little head-bashing on occasion. (Ah, you puzzle-solvers are with me, I can feel it.) This is obviously about vulnerability and brain injury. Very good. I did not recognize this until I just wrote it down.

Take Bosnia, Croatia, and Serbia for instance. I lived in Belgrade for a few months in the early '60s, as a teen. It was clear even then to a political neophyte like me that these tribes of people, feudally based and clan-oriented, were only biding their time until the Soviets left (as the Nazis had before them) and resume the pressing business at hand: killing each other, as they had for centuries. And for what? Sunflowers, pumpkins, corn, pigs, and migrating storks?

Cleansing what? Holocaust all over again. What did they learn from the Nazis? Or are they just passing it along? The whole thing is sick. And where did they get all those guns, anyway? Someone is bankrolling this deal. So I worry, about things I understand and things I do not. I worry about events I cannot control. Our foreign-policy mechanism is so broken.

There is, above all, a heightened suggestibility operating here and an accompanying reduction in immunity. The threatening, the scary, the hurtful, and the painful: all out of my control. Feeling like random violence surrounds and threatens me. Who in the shopping mall has or could have a gun, is angry, and may open fire at any moment? How about the guy in the car next to me. Is there a gun on the seat? If I look, will that trigger his thread-thin response?

All this on a bad day. The fear, paranoia, worry, and overactive imagination are exhausting. These sorts of thoughts creep in when my guard is weak. From safe to unsafe world. From peace to turmoil. Friendship to bloodshed. Tranquility to personal holocaust. Peace of mind to shattered truce.

Life's uncertainties suddenly grow from an occasional ticker-tape reminder to a sports bar-sized big screen turned way up so you won't miss a thing over the dancing, drinking, and shouting in the foreground. (Yeah, you are probably right, no dancing in a sports bar. Not enough women. See how my imagination carries me off?)

When morning's first thought is of breast cancer, especially when I am ovulating, I begin the day frightened and exhausted. How can I put this worrying to rest, while remaining reasonably vigilant?

Worrying, in this heightened state, is a new part of me. I struggle with it. I am not used to this bombardment. I wish the Alcoholics Anonymous prayer about knowing the difference between what I can and cannot change would work.

My prayer: this is a healing phase of my ever-recovering brain. This, too, shall pass.

Quick Trick to Stop Ideation

With a great deal of practice, I developed a way to get the worrying thoughts to stop. (1) If the worrying happened while my eyes were closed, I would open my eyes, say *NO*, then close my eyes again. If the thoughts were still there, I would repeat the process. (2) If the worrying thoughts happened while my eyes were open, I would close my eyes, say *NO*, then open my eyes once more. I would repeat until success was reached. This approach, reinforced with EMDR, really works. Ask your psychotherapist for help learning this skill.

You may find that a similar system, or different word selection, works better. Feel free to send the worrying thoughts packing. They do not serve your peace of mind. (See the chapter "But What If......Ideation.")

You may also discover the tactic of acknowledging and accepting the feelings, then releasing them. Use this affirmation to assist the process: *God, I accept the greater good you have ready for me now. I let go of worry and doubt, for they have no place in my life. I recognize that these types of feelings create unnecessary stress in me, so I gladly let them go. As I let go, I open the way for unlimited good to come into my life.*

A medical evaluation is imperative when ideations take control of your thinking, and it feels like your thoughts are out of hand. See your doctor.

Anxiety and Free-Floating Anxiety

Sometimes depression occurs with an overlay of anxiety. Sometimes you can tell what the anxiety is about, and frequently it is random, arbitrary, or "free-floating." Perhaps there is a feeling of dread or impending catastrophe, but you have no idea where it comes from. Your body may be tense, or you may clench your fists in your sleep. Sounds like anxiety to me.

This journal entry speaks to the experience.

MARCH 4, 1992

Today there is this anxiety. No, it's been here for weeks. The jaw clenching, the arms asleep and fists clenched at night, the animated loud voice, the tension, the urgency, the inner struggle—why?

There is a deep breath that just will not come in. Exercise helps. But the effect wears off almost immediately. There is an urgency to plan/schedule/control the time that ticks by. The hot tub does not relax me. The herbs help me sleep like a rock, but there is no daily net effect. My mind is racing, driven by adrenaline. I have been eating medicinal doses of chocolate to calm down. My jaw feels clenched in a relaxed position.

Anxious over what? My bills are paid, my practice is fine, my boyfriend is wonderful, my body is getting stronger and slimmer. Oh sure, the house needs a new roof, but that's not it.

Is this the next step in the brain-healing game? Is there some transition that takes me through generic idiopathic anxiety now? I cry a lot lately. And it's not my period. I feel rushed, in a panic to "settle" things, to decide things, to get things organized. Then, on the next page, I am angry that my life has not become a bowl of cherries yet. That my special psychic powers haven't made *my* lottery numbers turn up.

My body is tense all the time. No words, no hugs, no kisses, no music, no massage, hot tub, or decadence can erase the tension. I feel caught. Wedged in. Stuck. Trapped. Out of control. Out of ideas. Out of hope. I feel unused-used. Ineffective. Broken. But not broken enough to look broken. I feel robbed, cheated, stripped of my magic, as though I have lost my gift. My sense of personal value has wandered off and can't seem to get back home.

I feel as if I have drifted off and cannot remember where I live. The more I try to recall that simple sliver of thought, the more I flounder, and the sadder I become. I feel sucked down into a whirlpool of disconnectedness. I feel as if I have wandered off, lost my shoes, my way, and my hope. I feel sad today.

The good news is that it's physiologically impossible to be relaxed and anxious at the same time. Ask your biofeedback therapist to help you develop your relaxation response so that you can have a tool to handle uncontrolled anxiety.

Every ounce of energy you use up on anxiety takes away from your energy to think. Breathe and relax.

Depression and Physical Pain

If you sustained physical injury along with your brain injury, the simple act of coping with pain can also contribute to depression. It can also contribute to your fatigue. Dealing with pain takes tremendous energy. Even a persistent pain as light as a mild headache can affect your daily energy supply. (See the chapter "Physical.")

Physical pain can also take an emotional toll on your energy. (See the chapter "Emotions and Denial.") Ask your doctor about any medication that you are taking for pain. Some pain medications contribute to depression. Ask about side effects.

The New Lump on the Couch

Depression can lead to inactivity. That new lump on the couch could be you. With the help of your support system, arrange to engage in physical activity every day. Just 10 minutes a day will keep your body juices flowing. A walk around the block is a good start. (See the chapter "Support Systems" to learn how to ask for support and get a walking partner. Shop for or rent an easy exercise video. Every little bit helps get those feel-good endorphins flowing again.)

The Cloud Will Lift

The good news is that the cloud of depression gently begins to lift for most people as the healing process progresses. However, be forewarned that relapse will occur if you become too rambunctious in your recovery. Depression lifts gradually, and its lifting is not always consistent with the pace of the rest of the process. Don't party just yet.

Depression will often revisit you during a refueling period of your energy supply. A depression occurrence may surprise you if you have become used to brighter days. Understanding it will help you through the episode and not impede your overall progress.

This journal entry discusses a time of refueling. By then, I had discovered the value of quiet time.

MAY 12, 1992

> The depression now comes as a surprise, a feeling of wanting to hide, to go sit in front of the TV and let the electrical entertainment create a space for me to hide in. A space of nonaccountability, a risk-free hide-out, a place of quiet, a place of no demands. I cannot make mistakes in front of the TV. No one will tell, no one *can* tell. It's a refuge. Interestingly, I find myself defocused in front of the tube. Certainly it is not the content of the programming but the space it provides that is the essence of the moment. There are times when I need to un-be. To be exquisitely in time.

Summary

Depression is a serious symptom in your healing process. Learn by paying attention to your thoughts, feelings, and emotions. Treating depression appropriately can facilitate your recovery immensely. Discuss your sadness with your healthcare providers. They are in a better position to evaluate your depressive mood than you are.

39

But What if . . . Ideations

Your imagination may become overactive. As a result of anxiety, depression, and a changed perception of vulnerability, your brain may go off on tangents. At first it may feel that you have no control over what is known as "ideation."

Ideation creatively and enthusiastically answers the question "but what if?" Let's say you are standing at a crosswalk. There is a big truck coming down the street. There is a child across the street, waiting to cross also. "But what if" the kid goes into the crosswalk, the truck doesn't stop, the truck hits the kid? Well, I'd get the license of the truck, hold the dying kid in my arms, tell someone to call 911, administer CPR, get blood all over my clothes, and end up having to go home to change before continuing with my day.

All that, and you were just crossing the street. (But now your pulse is elevated, adrenaline kicks in, and you have a headache.)

Overactive imagination can kidnap a significant portion of your brain-functioning energy. This chapter will help you understand and direct your ideation episodes.

Your Launching Imagination

Your active imagination loves to run optional stories that result in worst-case scenario outcomes. These story endings have a life of their own, and they take an amazing amount of your brain's time and energy. You may also think you are really going nuts, to boot.

To this, I remind myself: No need to practice or review potential outcomes. If the time comes, I will know what to do.

Instant Empathy

The path toward ideation begins with instant empathy. Brain injury takes energy away from the brain's ability to discern and filter bits of information and thought. So the thought processes go straight to "what if this were happening to me" with no checks and balances.

Making dinner? What if I cut myself chopping onions? I'm alone in the house. The car is a stick shift. I can't drive. No neighbors are home. Where is my insurance card? How far is it to the hospital? Should I wrap my finger up in a towel and try to get there anyway? Maybe I could call a taxi. Then I would just get blood on the phone book. What if I pass out from the pain?

What if I just chopped this onion and sautéed it? ("I will know what to do.")

Ideation Run Amok

Ideation is amok to begin with. Your brain has plenty to do without adding fearful, panicky, scary, blood-and-guts cartoons to the menu. Ideation is a side effect of depression and will decrease as the depression decreases. Ruminations are also considered in this category, when thoughts go round and round without resolution.

Ideation can be a facet of depression. With depression as a reasonable and secondary response to brain injury, antidepressants may assist in ideation relief. Also consider that ideation can simply be a symptom of low-energy reserves unable to sort for viable thoughts.

If your ideations contain really serious thoughts, such as self-inflicted harm or violent harm to others, TELL YOUR HEALTHCARE PROFESSIONAL.

What to Do

After having about a year of run-on ideation, it occurred to me that I did not appreciate the extra adrenaline and scary stories I was telling myself. I set about figuring out how to make them stop.

I realized that sometimes the ideations occurred when my eyes were closed and sometimes when my eyes were open. I settled upon a plan that worked for me almost every time.

Just Say No

If the "what ifs" came when my eyes were closed, I would open my eyes and observe the reality around me. Either out loud or silently, I spoke the word "NO." Usually by the second "NO," the ideation was gone.

Conversely, if the ideations were a daydream with eyes open, I would shut my eyes, repeat "NO," and usually obtain success by the second repetition.

As the years have progressed, this technique generally works on the first attempt. EMDR worked to successfully reinforce the pattern.

Saying "NO" worked for me. It will be great to discover what you come up with to chase those silly stories out of your head. (See "Limbic Rage.")

DECEMBER 31, 1993: TAKE CONTROL OF HIT-AND-RUN IDEATION

Overwhelming, instant rageful mood. One minute happy as a clam. Next minute an uncontrollable urge to sweep all the kitchen counter dishes onto the floor. Where does this hit-and-run mood come from?

Many times this cloak of upset has settled upon me over the years, and every time I have wept, stomped around, slammed doors, thrown a few undamageable objects about, kicked a hole in the garage door, splattered food in the kitchen, screamed at the top of my voice, or cried inconsolably most of the night.

It has never been fun. I'm not proud of this behavior in the least, but have felt the prisoner of my thoughts. Perhaps another lovely quirk of the Brain Injury?

Until the other day. After a perfectly average evening, I walked into the kitchen to assemble and ingest my nightly vitamins. All of a sudden, the overwhelming rage swept over me. I saw myself beginning to reach for a heavily stacked counter of dirty dishes, when my mind said "NO." This voice inside me, a small pleading earnest voice said, "I don't want to do this episode."

Standing by the vitamins, hands on the counter, flannel nightgown in sweat, heaving and sobbing shoulders, tears running, breath halted, and shudders of emotion shaking my body, I blinked at the imaginary scene of kitchen chaos and I said "NO."

"I don't want to feel this way anymore." I called for my husband to hold me, then I blinked again and repeated the command "NO." My legs were jerking, I was sobbing but determined........Within 15 minutes all the symptoms of the episode dissolved. The relief was amazing to me. The emotional cloak conquered.

Most importantly, however, was the sense of empowerment at having sent away a debilitating ideation episode, which could have easily lasted hours. I was also empowered with the knowledge that this action could be repeated again when needed. And that I had recognized its onset. Knowing that it worked even once offers hope, strength, and a sense of reclaiming one's center of self.

The center of self can be sadly and tragically harmed by a brain injury. Self-image is a precious commodity, and during the journey on the long road to rediscovery of self, the brain-injured person deserves all the support and strength-building experiences possible. "Taking control" holds immeasurable value in this process.

Summary

Ideations, or the "what ifs," can be very distressing, draining, and frightening. Ideations drain energy. If ideation happens to you, notify your therapist. Over time, these episodes should diminish, along with properly treated depression. If ideations do not decrease, or if your thoughts turn self-destructive, tell your healthcare provider immediately. It is not healthy or supportive for you to live with this alone. Seek help.

40

Anger and Forgiveness

When you are an accident victim, the experience changes who you are and how you relate to your environment: emotions run deep. Anger may be the only emotion on your mind, whereas forgiveness may be the farthest.

This chapter looks at anger toward yourself and others and forgiveness of yourself and others. Here we talk about the fast track to getting on with your life. Pay attention.

Anger and Rage

When you have been hurt in an accident, someone or something is to blame. At least, that is what your mind tells you. Someone or something did this to you. AND YOU HATE THEM! It could be the car manufacturer, the drunk driver, the fogged windshield, or the guy on the bicycle or the ice on the sidewalk. But it was definitely someone else's fault.

And your life is messed up forever. Someone has to pay.

Who Is Responsible?

In many cases, there are clear provocateurs in the situation. Drunk driver runs a red light, and WHAMO!, you're on your way to the hospital.

In other cases, the sidewalk suddenly has gravel on it, or you come to a curve and your bicycle tires lose their traction. WHAMO!, you're on your way to the hospital.

Our litigious society pivots on fault and blame. Sometimes there is no clear source of the fault. Sometimes your judgment and the timing of the universe simply coordinate poorly.

The Anger Is Real

No matter how you got your brain injury, your anger about your present circumstances is genuine. Anger about the loss of your capacity, productivity, energy, and ability to be your previous self is very real. You have a right to be angry.

Hating Yourself

That anger is equally as real when it is turned inward upon yourself. How could this have happened to me? Why did I let this happen? Just three seconds either side of this moment and I would be fine. I hate what has happened to me. I hate this existence. I hate myself.

Anger directed inwardly is very destructive and demands a tremendous portion of your energy pie. It is normal to pass through a phase of self-bashing along the healing process trail. It is not healthy to dwell on it.

Forgiveness

The way out of the loop of anger is through forgiveness.

First of all, forgive the other party involved, if there is one. (Emotionally, but not necessarily legally. Ask your attorney.) Secondly, forgive the circumstances of the incident. Thirdly, forgive yourself for the losses you suffered in the accident. No argument. Just forgive. Let it go.

At Least Consider the Possibility of Forgiveness

If forgiveness is too much to ask just now, then at least be willing to picture and imagine yourself considering the possibility of forgiveness at some future time. Even this small thought will relieve some emotional pressure for you.

Another Important Consideration

At times, with brain injury, volatile issues in your life that had been previously contained and managed in your healthy psyche are suddenly too powerful for your limited energy reserve to inhibit. Old issues that you thought were resolved or at least contained may resurface.

When old issues recur, know that you do not have the energy reserve to resolve them now. Make allowances for these resurfaced issues. Alert your therapist to the issues. Your therapist is trained to devise a temporary containment strategy for you, until you have the necessary energy reserve to address them.

FEBRUARY 12, 1996: I'LL FOREVER HAVE A BRAIN INJURY

For all of the therapy, for all of the improvement, for all the ways life will get better or different or easier, the truth is I will always have a brain injury. With any luck at all, this will not be true for everyone who has suffered so. Some of you will be fully restored, and your memory of this healing time will fade with the years.

For some of us there will always be lingering remnants. Even though I can word process on my computer, I remain seriously challenged when it comes to putting numerical information on the Quicken bookkeeping system. The refocus-defocus-refocus progression coupled with sequential numbers overloads me and reduces my work to hunt and peck. I agonize over it. I stand before the high wall that reads: Things That Will Not Get Better.

There are other symptoms. Unannounced emotional fatigue crops up, although I must say in my own defense that the stress has to get pretty high before I crumble. And the crumbling is not as severe as it was a few years ago. The fact that it still happens saddens and angers me. I get this chapter out and read it again.

Summary

Acknowledge the many sides of anger and the potential for the healing effects of forgiveness. Consult a psychotherapist when anger issues occur or if old issues resurface. There is an appropriate time to proceed with a sufficient amount of anger work to effect forgiveness and progress. This is the real work. Ready when you are.

New therapy techniques like Somatic Experiencing are particularly effective with trauma resolution, old and repressed trauma issues and body pain associated with anger. Consider a therapist with this adjunct training.

41

Self-Esteem

How you see yourself, hold yourself, and present yourself to your environment are all vital to your recovery. The exploration of the "New You" will reveal your emerging identity and adapt it in the most functional and useful ways.

Some brain-injured people experience temporary personality changes, whereas others sustain permanent ones. These changes may be as minor as laughing more loudly at jokes or as significant as occupational changes from technical to artistic aptitude or vice versa.

This chapter will demonstrate a pathway to self-love, self-acceptance, and increased confidence and self-esteem.

Self-esteem, and the recovery thereof, is at the core of minor brain injury. When we falter, our confidence is deeply shaken. Self-acceptance wavers. Self-respect is in question. Self-love is out of the question. Internal, psychological underpinnings shift, and we may not know where they have gone. There is a "New You" emerging. It might feel like an arranged marriage. Who is this person, and how do I get to know her, let alone love her and have a happy life?

A hyperawareness of personal deficit contributes to a loss of self-esteem. You know what is missing. Here is something you need to know.

What you notice as deficit is how most people are in general. Can't remember a name, forget how to get across town, forget a birthday? Common to others, unthinkable to you. Now you do it and it's an almost unforgivable error. You lament aloud and people look at you like you are repeating the status quo.

But it's not *your* status quo. Your personal gauge is unfamiliar with these errors. How do you reconcile this behavior that you once judged in others and now are appalled by in your own life and mind? How to comprehend and deal as you judge?

— *G. Denton*

Confidence

Self-confidence can be eaten away slowly or ripped off in chunks. Either way, it is taxing to rebuild your confidence, especially when depression has taken its energy-depleting toll. It is vital to build your confidence, remind yourself that you are competent, and seek proof of confidence. To retrieve my confidence, I left town and went to hang out with strangers. I wanted to satisfy myself that I could manage a professional situation with people who didn't love me. I was looking for an unbiased opinion.

So, off to Moab, Utah, to the Pack Creek Ranch. The Canyonlands Field Institute was offering a seminar called "Desert Writers." This was my ideal getaway.

NOVEMBER 6, 1992

Seven hours in the car headed west, listening to motivational tapes all the way, directing the speaker's style, noting where he "borrowed" from more famous people (giving no credit due), noting his "reading" not "feeling" styles. It lets my mind wander as all good "mental confusion styles" will allow/promote.

Off to Utah; such a great place to think. A wondrous place to be still. A large, open and stunningly beautiful place to find the answers clattering around inside one's head or heart. Trying to discipline the two. Trying to shut up the head long enough to zero in on desire, passion. Why have I come here? The question flies across my mind quietly like a jet high overhead.

Why? The head answers: to get my confidence back. As if a simple act like driving over two snowy mountain passes, guzzling a thermos of cappuccino hot chocolate, munching a fresh Delicious apple from Colorado's Western Slope, and wolfing three cranberry muffins would do the trick. Not to mention the gas and nature stops and one brief pause to wash the mud from the headlights. The prolonged winter twilight brings out more than the requisite throng of highway deer coming to munch the abundant weeds and grasses that form the dried floral hedge illuminated by our intrusive headlights through the peaceful, crisp evening air. As if this simple act were a rite of passage to "the cure." As if the journey qualified one for presence near the magical place one procured this elusive puzzle piece.

Confidence. Where have I mislaid the confidence, as if the car keys have mysteriously been transported to my left pocket, where I would not look? Of course, I had them the whole time. Just can't grab them right now.

Yet confidence seems to hold me back. Am I seeking validation that my brain works again? From professionals? People I don't even know? Seven pavement-pounding hours from home? Yes.

Or did I just need the privacy that the driving allows? After all, everyone knows it's the journey, not the destination, that counts.

Yeah, yeah, my head chimes in. But facts are facts. Your brain isn't totally back yet. You know you still slur words and misspell and blank out. Yes, my heart replies, but she's still talented, functional and covers up well.

A piece of me sinks when I hear about "covering up." It's less immortal somehow. Flawed, not in an endearing way. Somehow I emerged different and see myself settling for less. The internal safety gauge seems stuck on "over-vigilant." But I'm healed now. I want to go out and play. The gauge kicks in the message, sends out the hormones and I turn on the TV and sit in safety. Well, thanks for the protection but enough already. I want my life back. The risk-taking part, the adventure, the glow.

I seize the piece that insists "I can, I must, I will" by the throat and demand action. Does that come from me? Do I dare? My heart beats "yes" and cheers me on. Confidence isn't in the dictionary between condoms and confetti. Not under the Christmas tree, nor under the hood of your car (in most cases) and not at the end of the rainbow.

It's there to grab, materializing only after the hand is extended. Appearing magically to fill the outstretched fingers. A response to passion exploded into the void; a baton firmly slapped into your palm. The fingers perform the final task, wrap around, hold on, get moving.

Utah is a big, open, dry, and silent place. If I lived here, I'd get my cruise control fixed. It's of little use in Colorado. Mostly I crack my knee on it. It's always good to come home. And I refreshed that all-important long-haul-driving skill of switching feet on the accelerator with a truck up my tailpipe and bunnies in the road. Rites of passage are clearly tailored.

Self-acceptance, self-love, and self-respect are integral to this process of regaining self-esteem. These terms are practically interchangeable. Work with the term that best matches how you feel or believe, the one that offers the most direct path to restored confidence.

Reality Check

It may be very helpful for you to seek professional support to obtain a reality check of your psychological status. Finding out if you are perceiving the world realistically is a great starting place. Find out if you are acting and reacting appropriately to your environment. Are you truly adjusting to your present reality? It is essential to perceive and understand your circumstances. It is one thing to understand and to respond in an awkward manner. It is quite another matter to misperceive your environment.

Psychotherapy is a valuable tool for checking your reality. However, be aware of the risks of being misdiagnosed by a therapist unfamiliar with brain-injury recovery. Keep your boundaries with your therapist. State your purpose and the length of time you wish to be seen. Be cautious of medications meant for depression, which may not apply to you. If it helps you, take a friend to your session. Remember, with therapy it is you who should experience changes or support. Keep looking if your first therapist seems inappropriate or unfamiliar with your condition. Finding someone who focuses on clients with mild brain injuries will generally give you a head start on this venture. Remind your therapist that your boundary issues are injury related to energy and disinhibition.

The New You: Adventures in Discovery

I still remember the day I got my results back from the neuropsychological evaluation. The neuropsychologist informed me that I had sustained some damage to my brain through impact and torque, and additional damage from oxygen deprivation. One result of this could be that I may become disinhibited in my social behavior. (See "The Beard Butcher of Boulder.")

Well, since I was a hot tub, mud bath, any excuse for a costume, closet full of silly hats kind of gal to begin with, I surmised that this news could be trouble. And, so far, it has been. The New Me laughs out loud more, acts on impulse more, leaves tact behind on occasion, and lives a bit more spontaneously.

Embarrassing for me. On the other hand, lots of shrinks charge bundles of money to tell people to go forth and do these very things to relieve stress in their lives.

So, it was new for me and embarrassing at times. But are these behaviors bad, on balance? This is where the reality check comes in. A behavior might be different to you and cause deep chagrin, but is it really *bad* behavior? It might just be the New You introducing herself with humor.

So fasten your seat belts kids, this will be a wild and bumpy ride. The more you treat it like an adventure, the more you discover about yourself. Remember, if this were Disneyland, you'd be paying big bucks for a safety bar and some hair-blowing adventure. So step right up and claim a seat. The ride begins now.

The Ego

Issues of the self and identity are most important when we self-judge. Coupling the internal dialog of "I should be able to..." with the overwhelming embarrassment of long-term illness can devastate self-esteem. Our culture holds long-term illness as shameful. Particularly if you *look* fine, you have a difficult time being perceived as ill in this culture. You may even wish for a cast, a limp, a cane, something that identifies you as "in the healing process."

Mental illness is the most culturally baffling of illnesses and carries with it the most cultural shame. Reflected helplessness from the culture is too much to bear. Yet, *this is not mental illness* but, rather, a bruise that takes forever to resolve. Remember that you are not crazy. And that our culture could benefit from an attitude adjustment!

Self-Esteem

When coupled with the added stress of brain injury, fragile self-esteem is a heavy burden to carry. Women with PMS (premenstrual syndrome) are familiar with this experience. One little thing can set you off and take you places you would never choose to go in a balanced state of mind. Remember that you are fragile and should treat yourself gently. Gently. Treat yourself gently at all times. Your energy is fragile, your strength is fragile, your emotions and self-esteem are fragile. Any little thing may set you off. Learning to love even those challenging moments is the key to giving yourself the space and time to heal.

Body Image

Your body chemistry may get out of balance. Your weight may fluctuate. You may experience immune deficiencies and contract an opportunistic infection, allergy, rash, cold, sinus infection, sexually transmitted disease, or yeast infection such as Candida (intestinal yeast).

Everything in your body is connected. It may feel like your body has betrayed you. Sure my brain is hurt, but why mess with my body, too? From the holistic perspective, you are a whole being, and what happens to a part of your being happens to your entire being. So, when your brain slows down, your body responds accordingly.

I put on 25 pounds and contracted an intestinal yeast infection. I followed a special diet to get rid of the yeast. I was afraid of exercise and would burst into tears at the gym. I got skin rashes, bloating, swollen lymph glands, and raging hormones. It took two years just to get rid of the yeast. So hang in there.

This is what I was thinking one day in October, 1992.

Where to start? The insidious depression. The weight. The good intentions. The Candida diet. This holistic view gives me too much to focus on! I feel lazy, unmotivated, unmotivatible, embarrassed, and lethargic.

My body sneezes, rashes, holds onto weight in spite of my clean diet, wants to exercise and finds every excuse not to. Itches. I still garble my words and hesitate when I spell. Rats!

Lots of other things are still working though! My business is doing fine. Not great, but no pressure. Confidence is low. Things I used to do well, I feel reticent to resume.

The chaos seems gone. I'm more rested emotionally. It shows. But so does this 25 pounds.

Just today I felt slender on the inside. For the first time since I fell. Like some meaningful stretching was finally happening inside. The first inkling of inner self-esteem. I felt graceful and slinky inside. It feels great. It's a sign I've been looking for. And a relief.

Rebuilding self-esteem without chaos and frantic life scheduling. Finally! Making choices that feed the new me.

Self-Judgment and Expectation

What are your expectations? Do you anticipate more than is reasonable or timely? Have you given yourself a schedule for recovery that satisfies your internal judge but ignores your body? Have you created an artificial standard that is more stringent than the goals you set before your injury? Notice how low self-esteem and self-anger play in on this calculation. Recovery is a reasonable goal. Over-achieving to attain recovery slows your pathway to success and throws in a few extra lashes to remind you of your pain. "The floggings will continue until the healing is complete." Think about it while you read this next journal comment. Sometimes, the slower you go, the sooner you reach your destination.

> Expectation. Shall I cast off that extra cloak of expectation—that need to over-satisfy, overproduce, overdo in order to feel at an even keel with the world? The truth is, the world isn't concerned about my keel. So if I backed off myself, added a little breathing room, a little extra floor space, my world would be roomier and I could take unmonitored deep breaths. The next veil is lifted. No more overtime for the judge. In fact, half time might be better. I hear the audience—fire the judge! We don't need no stinking judges!
>
> How would life be without that extra judgment looming over the left shoulder? Probably leave more room for the guardian angels to play. And my shoulders would weigh less.
>
> For an overachiever, it's the hardest part of the recovery plan.

Enthusiasm

There is a ratty looking sticky note in this file that reads

Enthusiasm = Self-esteem:

I love myself enough to risk sharing my inner passion.

To me this means it is important to tell the truth of my needs, regardless of what that might look like to me or anyone else. One of the puzzle pieces of self-esteem recovery is to state what you are about and to ask yourself and others for what you want.

Summary

I support you in the return of your self-esteem, with your starts and fits, with or without smooth rendition, in whatever form it arrives and whatever the temporary appearance. Enthusiasm is a sure sign that self-esteem is rearing its confident head. You are on a path walked by many. You are among friends. Blurt out your needs. Head high.

42

Déjà Vu

A great many people who have experienced mild brain injury acquire the ability to anticipate or perceive events before they happen or to feel familiar in an unfamiliar situation, as if they have "done it before." The feeling of deja vu, and other heightened experiences of active intuition, ESP (extra sensory perception), or psychic or paranormal episodes, are a common occurrence after brain injury.

This is a take it or leave it chapter that explores the new skill of "knowing," perceiving, or experiencing information that can't be proven. It acknowledges the presence of paranormal events, or the increase in same, for the brain injured. In the event of this occurrence during your recovery, we hope the following insights are of use. It describes some kinds of events or phenomena that are most common with this new skill. It helps you understand this heightened state of awareness. If you have never before experienced deja vu, it helps dispel the myths and lets you explore rather than fear the events. For many, it expands spiritual awareness or a sense of religious presence or inner peace.

Being Psychic

There are two kinds of people in the world: those who believe in psychic ability and those who do not. There are also those who, after a brain injury, come to experience paranormal activity whether or not they previously believed in it. The trick is to let go of your judgments about paranormal behavior. Psychic ability is not good, bad, weird, evil, the work of the underworld, or a plot to control your mind from outer space. It is a phenomenon. It may happen to you whether or not you believe in it.

If you were not aware of paranormal knowledge before your accident, it can be an unexpected, startling, surprising, disturbing, or serendipitous experience. You can suppress it, ignore it, enjoy it, judge it, or exercise it.

You may develop a feeling of "knowing." You may know something that you cannot know, based upon empiric data. You may receive information that you cannot receive through normal means. This may be as simple as knowing that your spouse is almost home. You picture her driving through the neighborhood. You "feel" her getting closer to the house. You look out the window, and, no surprise to you, she pulls up.

The phone rings. You know who it is. You know, not because you asked him to call. You know because the information that he was calling reached you before the phone rang. Or you know because you were thinking of him and asking in your mind for him to call. He called.

Have you answered the door because you felt someone was approaching your home? The Japanese have a name for this sense of proximity: shibumi. It expresses that you have a relationship with the people and objects in your general vicinity and that you sense their presence and proximity to you.

Please note that paranormal incidents, like other experiences outlined in this book, may or may not be a part of your experience.

Your Radar Just Got Better

Think about how our relatives communicated in ancient times. Consider the traditions of civilizations long before our time that relied upon extrasensory communication in their daily lives and in their spiritual lives.

Now, with your brain injury, you have been sent deep into your old brain, which is calling the shots. Could it be that the old cell memory of this lost skill is surfacing? Has our noisy, complicated society robbed us of this ancient ability? Has your injury given you a path back to this old skill? Could be.

Most importantly, you have added a most intriguing skill at a time when other skills have been temporarily withheld. Let it be. Enjoy the information.

Spiritual Awareness

You may experience an increased interest in spiritual matters. You may experience an awakening to spiritual matters for which you held no previous interest. This may be a general awakening to a higher power, a heightened sense of awareness of the general natural beauty of the earth, or a strong epiphany or rebirth of your previously held religious convictions.

Many people, but certainly not all, experience a change in their interest in a power outside or inside themselves. And, of course, this may not happen.

If, in the course of your accident, you experienced a "near death," your sense of spiritual awareness may be likewise heightened. Many times, a near-death experience will bring with it additional paranormal insights and abilities. Along with that may come spiritual, moral, or ethical revelations, bringing the person to live life from a differently informed base of understanding.

Near-death experiences range from the traditional "tunnel of white light," to the life of the person flashing before her, to voices and conversations, or to an overwhelming sense of peace and contentment. Each event is unique to the individual, and fascinating to hear.

JUNE 28, 1991: NEAR DEATH

I have walked up to the door of heaven, knocked, and gone unanswered. I have been sent back to complete my work in this life. I feel compelled that my life must now be somehow different. Is this a real, a normal feeling? That since I came back it was for a reason?

And must that reason be big? Profound? A mission somehow? Or can I just lower my cholesterol, exercise more, and find a good life companion?

Was I spared? Saved? Brought back? Or a fortunate child of the '90s, a gift of modern science. In any other century, I would have died. Except In-line skates weren't invented yet. Small detail.

So how am I to be different? Throughout this recovery I watch as certain parts of me heal, return, jump-start, or wobble back. Before I was just sleepy, weak, and unconnected. Now, my brain and eyes are working a little too much to be a fully contented inmate. We've passed through the first few energy centers and more of me remembers who I am (was).

Déjà Vu and the Analytical Brain

If your mind is used to being very linear, pragmatic, and logical, this chapter may be most valuable to you. Especially if anything that is "nonlinear" is unacceptable, nonsensical, illogical, or out of control.

When a left-brain thinker experiences a brain injury, there are instances of a shift to right-brain dominance that may include such nonlinear explorations as psychic premonition, feelings of deja vu, or cognitive reception of unsolicited information.

A useful way to handle that experience is to chalk it up to a "piece of the new you" over which you have no control. It is not to be feared, judged, or sent packing. You just may have a new piece of radar installed that gives you random information. You can choose to observe it or not, use it or not, explore it or not. Your motherboard is running new software. Be not afraid.

The Paranormal

The story about climbing in Rocky Mountain National Park over July 4th offers a glimpse into the paranormal. Find the journal entry in the chapter "Risk and Initiation," and read it with new eyes.

Intuition and Premonition

Even for people like me, who have a heightened sense of intuition and long ago stopped counting the number of coincidences in our lives, there are those Twilight Zone moments when the familiar notes of the "do-do-do-do" melody slip in and offer their unsolicited gift.

> Staring off into space into the far reaches of my desk, I spied a clipping I had taped there some seven months ago. Omarr Reads the Stars.
>
> I had cut this one out because it seemed propitious at the time. "You won't be standing still. Emphasis on travel, learning experience, communication, discovery of 'soul mate.' Previous limitations no longer apply."
>
> The soul mate part I circled in red ink. Hadn't seen any pronouncements like that from Omarr in years. Soul mate had a nice ring to it, so up it went.
>
> Then I fell seven days later, and my mind and life have been preoccupied with other things.
>
> Until yesterday, when I glanced at it again. And saw that the date was May 20, 1991. Dan's birthday. In two years, he would be my husband.
>
> What did you wish for just before you blew out your candles?

Summary

This "take it or leave it" chapter introduces the concept of an increased or newly installed skill known as extra sensory awareness. It is a potential byproduct acquired with brain injury. It serves at your pleasure.

Resources

"Refuse to let other people define your boundaries and enforce your limitations. The seeds of greatness are on the inside of you and they are waiting to be birthed. Hold onto your flexibility and sense of humor. You will need it on the ride of life! It is seldom a smooth ride but you can be the driver. There will be falls along the way, but the difference between a success and a failure is choosing to get up one more time in whichever way you can.

There is a way out and we choose to define it. We do not need to be defined or limited by other peoples' boundaries. You hold the keys that unlock the door to your future. We are all changed by the things we see and the people we meet. Your opportunity is waiting. Go and meet it!"

Dr. Amy Price, 2007

Products

www.brainlash.com "Fieldguide to Brainlash," Audiotape by Gail L. Denton, PhD, an interview with the author. Offers additional information about living with brain injury. An ideal tape to offer friends, family, coworkers, attorney, and healthcare providers. It explains the experience of Brainlash and conserves your energy!

www.brainlash.com Earplugs

Brain Age   Cognitive brain-training game for a Nintendo.

Big Brain Academy   Cognitive brain-training games for a Nintendo.

Celestial Seasonings   "Ginkgo-Sharp Tea."

Colored Eye Glasses   (colored plastic: the four colors most commonly used: blue, gray, red, bright yellow can stabilize the printed page and keep the print from moving.) Available at many natural food stores.

www.eyelights.com   Eye light therapy glasses to activate the brain.

www.FranklinCovey.com   Franklin Day Planner: 1-800-654-1776

www.earplugstore.com   Earplugs

Rescue Remedy   A Bach Flower Essence, available at natural foods retailers.

Visigraph   A vision-evaluation tool. See Accelerated Performance.

www.vision3d.com   A website dedicated to eye therapy. It's free!

www.MyBrainTrainer.com   Cognitive brain training on your home computer.

www.tintavision.com   Tintavision

Treatment Modalities

Accelerated Performance,   Dr. Edvin Manniko, OD, 303-691-9128

www.brainmattersinc.com   Brain Matters, SPECT brain scan diagnostic

www.interactivemetronome.com   Therapy used to treat cognitive dysfunction

www.li-integratedmedical.com   Brain balance music

www.i-waveonline.com   Brain balance music

www.vision-therapy.com   Behavioral optometry

www.nora.cc   Neuro-Optometric Rehabilitation Association

www.neurofunction.com   Neurofeedback

www.ochslabs.com   Neurofeedback

www.sensorylearninginstitute.com   Sensory integration therapy

www.emerson.edu   Chronic pain info (Health Communications Resources)

www.optometrists.org   Optometrists Network—excellent vision info

www.amenclinic.com   Clinic associated with the book *Making A Good Brain Great*

www.youramazingbrain.org   Brain teasers

www.sharpbrains.com   Brain teasers

www.puzz.com   Brain teasers

www.puzzle.dse.nl   Brain teasers—click on the UK flag on the web site for the English version

www.sparksofgenius.com   Sparks of Genius—learning assessment tool

www.thelisteningprogram.com   The Listening Program—learning assessment tool

Organizations

www.theacpa.org   American Chronic Pain Association

www.AMTAmassage.org   American Massage Therapy Association

www.polaritytherapy.org   American Polarity Therapy Association

www.oep.org   Optometric Extension Program Foundation—behavioral optometry

www.healthy.net/associations/pa/oep/VISION.HTM

www.biac.org   Brain Injury Association of Colorado

www.biawa.org   Brain Injury Association of Washington. The most informative and helpful site! 1-206-621-8558

www.braingym.org   Brain Gym—educational kinesiology

www.thebrainmatters.org   American Academy of Neurology Foundation

www.neuroskills.com   Center for Neuro Skills and TBI Resource Guide

www.headinjury.com   Brain Injury Resource Center—excellent info site.

www.biausa.org   Brain Injury Association of America—local state sites are listed on this website.

www.nih.gov   National Institutes of Health—Rehabilitation of Persons with Traumatic Brain Injury Consensus Development Conference Statement, on the web or order a print at 1-888-644-2667

www.open.org   Northwest Neurodevelopment Training Center

www.healthtouch.com   Pain control info

www.spinalinjuryfoundation.org   The Spinal Injury Foundation

www.tbiguide.com   Traumatic Brain Injury Survival Guide 231-935-0388

www.upledger.com   Upledger Institute for Cranio-Sacral Therapy

www.Subtlebraininjury.com

www.biawa.org/links.htm

www.braintrain.com

www.brainconnection.com

www.abihelp.org

www.brainsource.com

www.cccv-ltd.com

www.biof.com/captainslog.html   Captain's Log, an online cognitive therapy choice

www.tbiresources.com

www.neurotraumaregistry.com

www.betsysupportpage.com

www.tbicommunity.org

www.webring.com

www.bindependent.com   Lifestyle products for independent living

www.tbimatters.org

www.novavision.com

www.braininjurysuccess.org

www.operation-helmet.org

www.ClaudiaOsborn.com

www.neurotherapies.com

www.neurotherapycenters.com

www.PlayAttention.com

Notes

1. M.L. Acimovic, M.A., et. al., *Energy Allocation in Mild Traumatic Brain Injury*, 1994.

2. *Trial Talk*, June 1992, Daniel A. Hoffman, M.D.

3. Mary Ann Keatley, Ph.D., personal interview.

4. Margaret Ayers, Head Injury Frontiers, 1987, p. 380.

5. Mary Lou Acimovic, M.A., C.C.C.

6. *The Brain: Fact, Function, Fantasy*, Northwest Neurodevelopment Training Center.

7. Dr. Rebecca Hutchins, O.D. and Dr. Edvin Manniko, O.D., for their guidance and information in the writing of the vision chapter. Personal communication.

8. Read "The Rosedale Diet," "Fantastic Voyage," "The Schwartzbein Principle," among others.

9. Giza and Hovda, 2000 and 2001 research.

Bibliography

The truth is, the science of Nature has been already too long made only a work of the brain and the fancy; It is now high time that is should return to the plainness and soundness of observations on material and obvious things.

Robert Hooke, 1665

Helpful Books

Amen, Daniel G., "Making a Good Brain Great, Fifteen Days to a Better Brain." 2005, ISBN 1-4000-8208-0.

Dennison, Paul E., and Gail E. Hargrove. "EK for Kids," Edu-Kinesthetics,

Il Chi Lee, "Brain Respiration, A Powerful Technique To Energize Your Brain," 1998, Han Mun Hwa Publishing, ISBN 89-86481-34-0.

Katz, Lawrence C., and Manning Rubin, "Keep Your Brain Alive," Workman Publishing, 1999.

Kurzweil, Ray, and Terry Grossman, "Fantastic Voyage: Live Long Enough to Live Forever," Rodale Press, 2004, ISBN 1-57954-954-3.

Larsen, Stephen, "The Healing Power of Neurofeedback: The Revolutionary LENS Technique for Restoring Optimal Brain Function. (See also: www.ochslabs.com, www.stonemountaincenter.com, www.neurotherapycenters.com.)

Ornstein, Robert, and David Sobel, "The Healing Brain, Breakthrough Discoveries About How The Brain Keeps Us Healthy," Touchstone Press, Simon and Schuster, 1987.

Osborn, Dr. Claudia, "Over My Head, A Doctor's Account of Head Injury from the Inside Looking Out." 1998, ISBN 0-9658750-0-8.

Richards, Byron J., "Mastering Leptin: The Leptin Diet; Solving Obesity and Preventing Disease," 2004, ISBN 0-9727121-1-9.

Rosedale, Ron, "The Rosedale Diet: Turn Off Your Hunger Switch," 2004, HarperCollins, ISBN 0-06-056572-1.

Schwarzbein, Diana, "The Schwarzbein Principle: The Truth About Losing Weight, Being Healthy and Feeling Younger," 1999. ISBN 1-55874-680-3.

Schwarzbein, Diana, "The Schwarzbein Principle II: The Transition," 2002, ISBN 1-55874-964-0.

Schwarzbein, Diana, "The Schwarzbein Principle: The Program," 2004, ISBN 0-7573-0227-0.

Willcox, Bradley J., et al, "The Okinawa Diet Plan: Get Leaner, Live Longer, and Never Feel Hungry," 2004, ISBN 1-4000-4953-9.

Wilson, James L, "Adrenal Fatigue: The 21st Century Stress Syndrome," 2001, ISBN 1-890572-15-2.

Useful Articles

Acimovic, Mary Lou, M.A. et.al., "Energy Allocation in Mild Traumatic Brain Injury," 1994.

Berne, Samuel A. "Visual Therapy for the Traumatic Brain-Injured," *Journal of Optometric Vision Development*, December 1990, Vol. 21.

Binder, L. M., "Persisting Symptoms After Mild Head Injury: A Review of the Post-Concussive Syndrome." *Journal of Clinical and Experimental Neuropsychology*, 1986, Vol.8, No. 4.

Donovan, E. M., "Coming to My Senses." *New Age Journal.*

Down, Richard, "An Insult to the Brain," *Discover*, Vital Signs, February 1994.

Hoffman, D. A., "Finally, Accurate Diagnosis and Quantification of Mild Closed Head Injury (with Implications for Treatment)," *Trial Talk*, June 1992.

McMahon B. T., and Flowers, S. M. "The High Cost of a Bump on the Head," *Business and Health,* Washington Business Group on Health.

Pollens, R. D., et al., "Beyond Cognition: Executive Functions in Closed Head Injury," *Cognitive Rehabilitation*, September/October, 1985.

Sierra, Bonita Infantino. "From the Patient's Point of View," *The Journal of Cognitive Rehabilitation*, September/October 1993.

Sweeney, J. E., "Non-impact Brain Injury: Grounds for Clinical Study of the Neuropsychological Effects of Acceleration Forces," *The Clinical Neuropsychologist*, 1992, Vol. 6, No.4.

Veach, Roger, "Minor Head Injury Equals Major Problems," *Trial Talk*, February 1989.

Weiner, Lowell B., Leslie Grant, and Alan Grant, "Monitoring Ocular Changes that Accompany Use of Dental Appliances and/or Osteopathic Cranio-sacral Manipulations in the Treatment of TMJ and Related Problems," *The Journal of Cranio-mandibular Practice*, July 1987, Vol. 5, No. 3.

Index

Note: Boldface numbers indicate illustrations.

CPSIA information can be obtained
at www.ICGtesting.com
Printed in the USA
FSOW03n1143101017
39735FS